CREATING
SANCTUARY

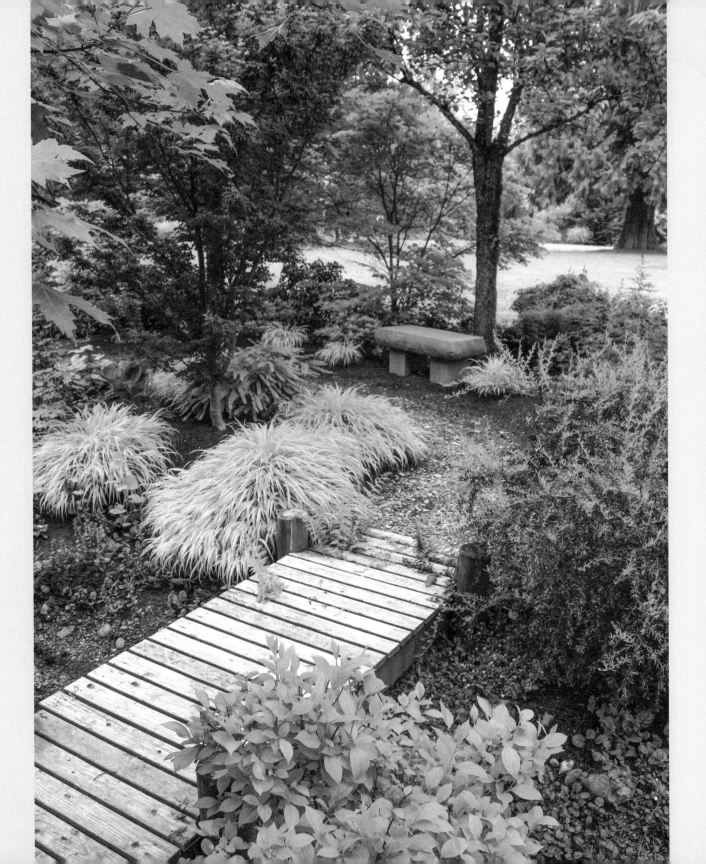

CREATING SANCTUARY

Sacred Garden Spaces, Plant-Based Medicine,
and Daily Practices to Achieve Happiness and Well-Being

by

JESSI BLOOM

with photos by SHAWN LINEHAN

Timber Press · Portland, Oregon

FRONTISPIECE A sanctuary you create in your own backyard can nourish your spiritual, emotional, and physical well-being by offering peacefulness, protection from a harsh world, and medicine for body and soul.

Published in 2018 by Timber Press, Inc.

The Haseltine Building
133 S.W. Second Avenue, Suite 450
Portland, Oregon 97204-3527
timberpress.com

Printed in China

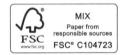

Text and cover design by Hillary Caudle

Library of Congress Cataloging-in-Publication Data

Names: Bloom, Jessi, author.
Title: Creating sanctuary: sacred garden spaces, plant-based medicine, and daily practices to achieve happiness and well-being / by Jessi Bloom; with photos by Shawn Linehan.
Description: Portland, Oregon: Timber Press, 2018. | Includes bibliographical references and index. |
Identifiers: LCCN 2018011961 (print) | LCCN 2018015769 (ebook) | ISBN 9781604698930 | ISBN 9781604697544 (pbk.)
Subjects: LCSH: Sanctuary gardens. | Gardens—Design. | Medicinal plants.
Classification: LCC SB454.3.S25 (ebook) | LCC SB454.3.S25 B56 2018 (print) | DDC 635.9--dc23
LC record available at https://lccn.loc.gov/2018011961

A catalog record for this book is also available from the British Library.

I dedicate this book to all of my teachers: the two-legged, the four-legged, the winged, the rooted, and my own spirit. I am forever grateful for the lessons I have learned from my experiences, and for the wisdom that's been shared.

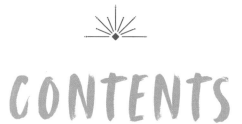

CONTENTS

14

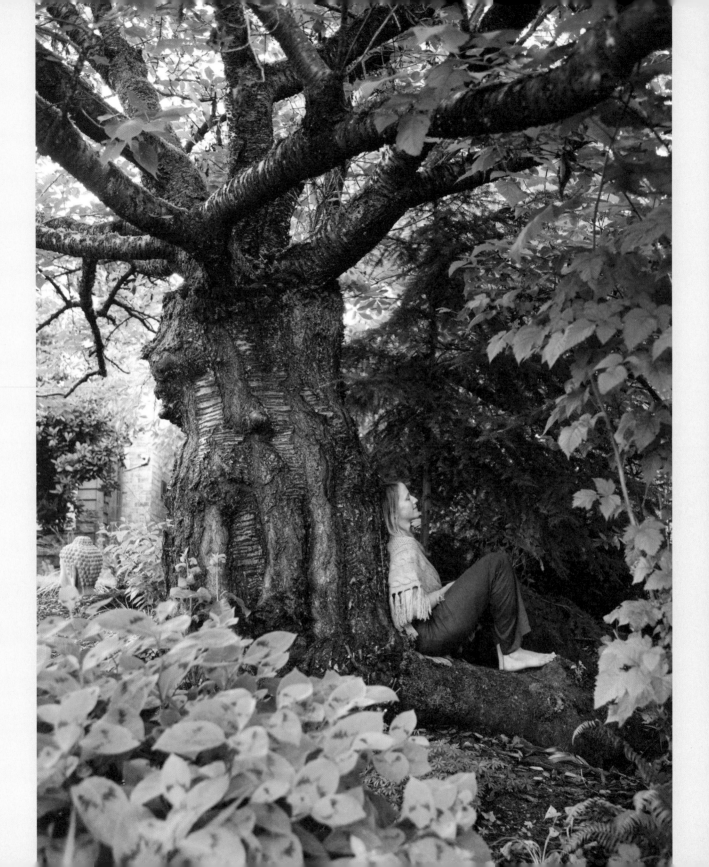

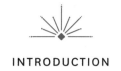

Coming Home To Yourself

"Within you, there is a stillness and a sanctuary to which you can retreat at any time and be yourself."

HERMAN HESSE, *SIDDHARTHA*

I find sanctuary sitting with Wanda, the elder cherry tree in my front yard.

We all need sanctuary. We need a place where we can feel safe, one that rejuvenates and refreshes us, somewhere we feel nourished and loved.

Many of us look for that sweet spot in the wildness of a distant national forest or park, the aisles of a high-priced grocery store, or a trendy exercise class. Often we look to connect to nature anywhere that has more plants than people, more wildlife than domesticated or controlled life. It may be our habit to get into a car and drive somewhere in hopes of becoming ourselves again, especially after a bad day or during a rough period. We acknowledge that when we eat better and exercise we feel good, and that the connections we find in nature help to restore our spirit, but what we overlook is how much of that we can find right in our own backyards. All of us can use our gardens, the earth, and spaces we inhabit

9

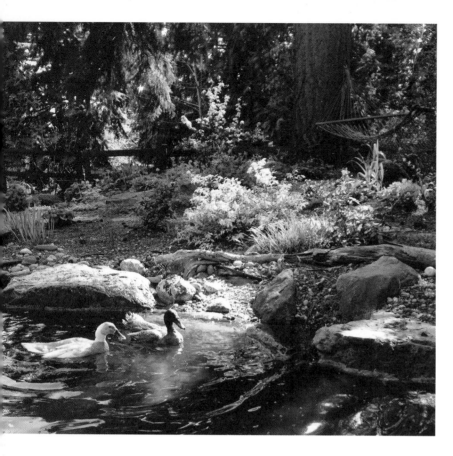

Being surrounded by harmonious elements and other life forms can be soothing to our nervous systems.

all around us, in the news, on social media, in our own neighborhoods. Stress mounts until it consumes us, and then Western medicine encourages us to treat illness with drugs that mask the symptoms so we can resume the same routine that caused the stress in the first place.

How do we change? How do we get out of this rut and practice self-care regularly? How do we effectively create a way of living that allows us to heal, feel restored, and find peace within ourselves? We can do this by incorporating what is good for us into our daily routines and shaping the environments we find ourselves in every day so they inspire us too.

I believe that nature is the best healer. When we remember that we *are* nature and when we take our place there as one species among countless other species, we feel nature's raw energy—water, wind, sun, sturdy trees, burgeoning blossoms—and are able to forget about our own worries for a little while. The life force that runs through our own bodies can resonate with all of nature's energy if we let it. But before we can, most of us have to learn to take care of our nervous systems and not to carry negative energy around in our bodies. By looking to nature, we can find simple ways to keep ourselves healthy. And when we take care of ourselves, our interactions with others improve, too, leading to overall societal well-being.

as our personal sanctuary. This book is about creating sanctuary, every day, wherever we find ourselves.

The busyness of our lives can often distract us from making time to find relaxation or peace, to ground ourselves, and to really evaluate where we are heading. There is cultural pressure to do more, to have more, and to push ourselves too hard. We tell ourselves that the tasks and to-do lists we create are more important than self-care and quiet reflection. We often take care of others' needs before our own, at the expense of our health: body, mind, and spirit. We see hardship and challenge

My intention in this book is to help you transform your life by caring for nature in the space you already have and learning to use its simple, powerful gifts effectively. I hope to

* help you find a deeper relationship with and connection to the land you inhabit—no matter the size—and with all of its beings and elements;

* share my love of plants and my knowledge of all they can offer us; and

* help you find sanctuary every day by incorporating simple, nature-based routines.

My own journey to find sanctuary has been a lifelong adventure. I grew up in a small rural community close to the woods in the foothills of the Cascade Mountains and with a view of the Salish Sea. My home was not always safe, however, nor were many of the people in my neighborhood. I would escape to the forest to find sanctuary, hiding there until I felt protected and whole. There, I could be me. Nature would hold me securely, letting me explore, learn, and feel supported.

My relationship with wild environments only grew stronger as I approached adulthood. My passion for nature expanded in defense of the sacredness I felt there. I wanted to protect and serve the resource that had kept me safe and

I have always been able to feel the life force inherent in plants as I have loved and studied them.

nourished in those early years of my life. I tended to plants in nurseries, harvested their seeds for ecological restoration, pruned them, loved them, studied them, and ultimately found myself in a successful career as a horticulturalist, environmentalist, and landscape designer. I was drawn to this path because I've always been able to feel the life force inherent in plants, animals, earth, water, and stone.

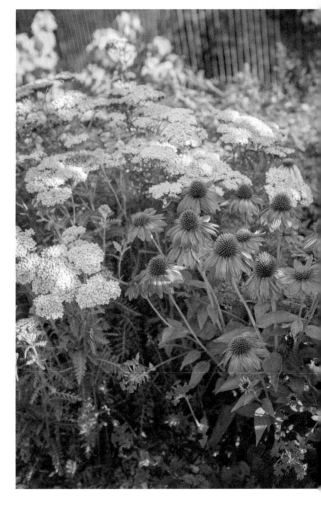

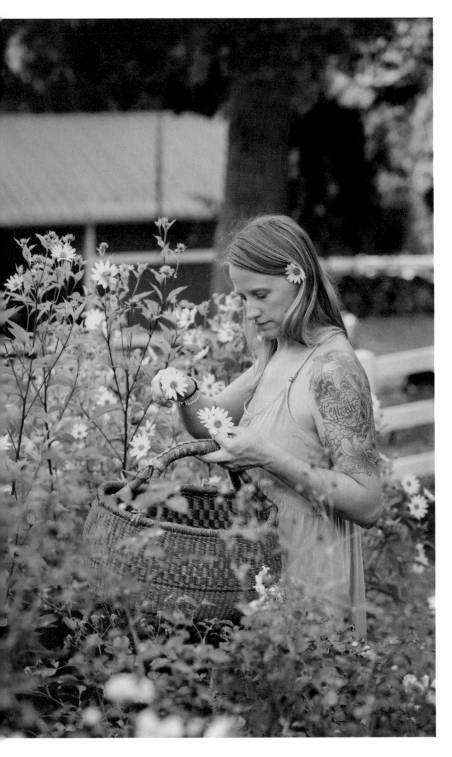

I often see myself as a connecting point between people and their own environments, an interpreter between humans and nature. My job has been to help people create sanctuary at home by developing and nurturing sacred spaces we shape together in their own gardens.

While my career was taking off, I was running a growing-too-fast business, raising two children, and volunteering in my community and industry to help with awareness and stronger environmental standards. Then came a tipping point. I simply ran out of energy. I had medical problems left and right. My body's systems were failing me; I had respiratory issues from carbon monoxide poisoning, I needed surgery for my kidneys, and toxic diagnostic scans wreaked havoc on the rest of my body. I saw numerous specialists but eventually realized that underlying these mechanical failures was my failure to nurture my own emotional and spiritual health.

Another turning point was getting divorced. Picking up pieces of my life after it had seemingly exploded forced me to slow down and adjust my lifestyle. I began to wonder what had happened. How had I become so focused on the

Harvesting plant medicine from my garden has been an important part of my own healing.

outside world that I had failed to create sanctuary in my own life, to take care of my own most basic needs? Suffering from post-traumatic stress disorder (PTSD), searching for healing on every level, I made a dramatic shift in my life, and my journey took a new course.

I looked far and wide and kept my mind open. I discovered powerful healing in the teachings and modalities of many other cultures. I was especially drawn to the way plants were used as medicine throughout time, so I began to seek out and connect the dots between different plant-based methods. Interestingly, I found many parallels between folk medicine and scientifically validated modern medical uses of plants. People have been using plants for healing from the beginning of our species and around the globe—and our collective knowledge about the healing power of plants somehow survived without all the communication systems we rely on today.

My garden—its plants and the animals that visited it—was my sacred space while I healed during a period of several years. My connection to the land kept me going. I knew it was time to shift my life to focus on self-care and to turn to nature for remedies. During this period, I began asking myself many questions: What helps us function well? What makes us happy? What keeps us stuck in destructive or unhealthy behavioral patterns? How can nature help us heal from trauma? How can we live the best life possible in harmony with the world around us? I decided to focus on helping people find better and more resilient ways to live in a world that seems increasingly complex and at times irreparably damaged and hostile.

Sanctuary is becoming more important than ever before. The surest way for us to be able to live in peace and to be happy is for us to create a place where we can be in harmony with the natural world and where we feel comfortable in our own skin. When we achieve this, we restore our bodies, minds, and souls.

You can find everyday sanctuary in any patch of land that brings you into proximity with nature—including your own backyard. Just as you can decorate an interior space in a way that suits you and makes you feel happy, you can create a garden to nourish your spiritual and emotional well-being. All land is sacred. All life is sacred. Therefore, anytime you infuse a space with positive intentions and honor the relationship you have with the life and energy inside that space, it can become an everyday sanctuary for you. This book will help guide you on that journey.

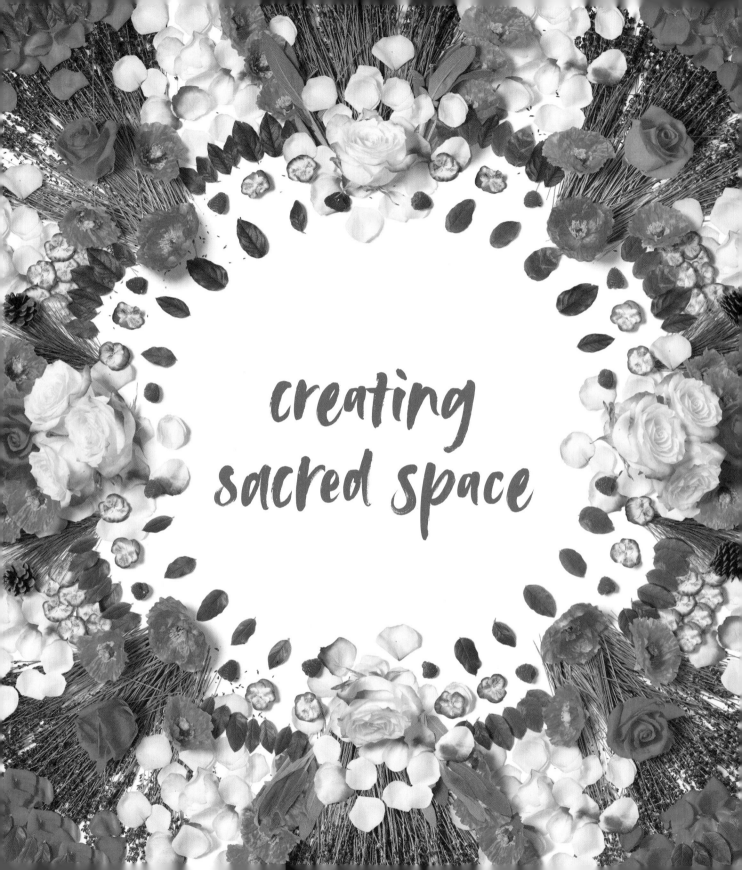

creating
sacred space

*"Your sacred space is where you can
find yourself again and again."*

JOSEPH CAMPBELL

◆

What is sacred space? What does it mean to create your own sacred space? What does it take to build your own sanctuary? How can a space you inhabit every day nurture your body, mind, and soul? No two people I've ever spoken to have had the same response when I've asked how they would define a sacred space, but most focus on themes of peacefulness, protection from a harsh world, and rejuvenation.

For me, a place that exemplifies sacred space is Orcas Island. It isn't too far from where I grew up, yet when I was a child my family never

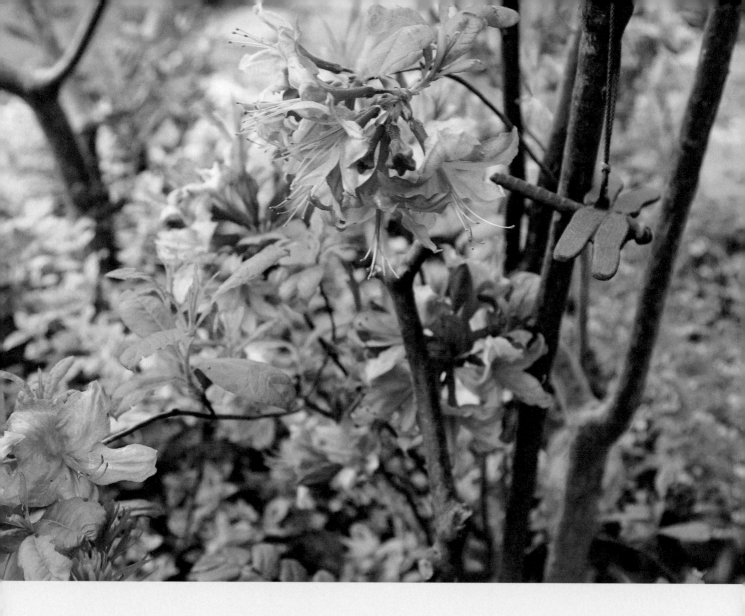

To create sacred space, we must start with our intentions. In the space pictured, creating beauty and honoring life (including insects) are the intentions.

visited due to the expense and time required to get there. As an adult, I took a boat there, and as soon as I set foot on the land I knew deep down it was special. I had spent much of my childhood exploring and foraging in the national forest land and the raw riverbeds flowing into the Salish Sea, and those places had resonated with me, but this island felt different. Every part of it spoke to me. Portions of it were truly wild, and even the areas that had been farmed or gardened had been cultivated with love and good stewardship. It was protected, and its inhabitants had prioritized honoring the land and looking ahead to the future. When the trip ended, I couldn't wait to plan my return—it was as if the island had spoken to me and awakened my soul to the sacredness of the earth. I wanted to be nowhere else.

I've been fortunate since then in being able to visit many sacred natural spaces—public and private, near and far, some thousands of years old and some just created. I've experienced everything from degraded ancestral sacred lands that had been covered in garbage to spaces treated with such regard that people were not even allowed to enter. At each, I tried to pay particular attention to the different ways they promoted human health and wellness. All the human-designed sanctuaries were founded with clear intentions, and their creators filled them with resources to support a vision or goal.

What I learned is that to determine what made a place so exquisite, I needed to look at the history in the soil, how the land was treated and cared for by the people who lived there, previously and now. What makes something sacred is at least partly how we treat it. This truth makes me ask myself why all land isn't treated as sacred and worthy of honor and respect. To my mind, stewardship of the earth has always been our most fundamental task in life. When we take care of the earth, it takes care of us. The three chapters that follow build on that understanding as they walk you through the process of designing and creating your sacred space.

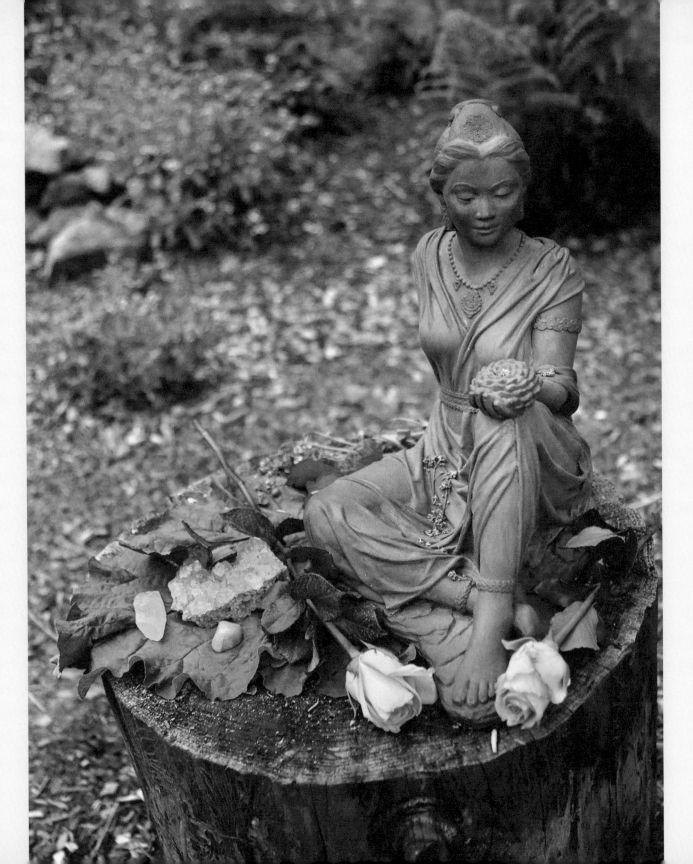

Envisioning Your Sanctuary

Sanctuary can look different for everyone. Here, a statue of Buddhist deity Kuan Yin graces the garden with a reminder of deep compassion and unconditional love.

When we are designing any space, we can have a lot of fun dreaming of the possibilities. I want to encourage you first to create a personalized definition of sanctuary. What do your spirit and your soul need?

This chapter will guide you in creating a plan that includes everything you think you could possibly want. A plan to create your own Eden, your own paradise. To create holy ground. To create whatever your heart desires. Creating such a plan often entails facing fears and anxiety, and ultimately looking at much deeper issues than just daydreaming about plants or putting together idea boards. How would you like to take care of the earth, and how would you like it to take care of you?

Defining your sanctuary starts with listening to the spirit already present in your own space. Every piece of land is different and has unique constraints and attributes. I believe as stewards of the land, we are to honor it first and foremost.

Then we can feel and envision what we need, want, and desire, and make sure this is in alignment with what the land needs in order to be cared for.

You might want to start a special notebook, journal, or binder for your sacred space exploration. Add to it as you open yourself to impressions that may form as you observe your land and your own relationship to it over a period of time, as your intentions and desires for the space become clearer, and as you gather inspiration from other places. Think of it as a place to dream and imagine.

Ethical Guidelines for Designing Sacred Spaces

The earth is alive, breathing and evolving, and all that she carries and supports forms a weave of complex ecosystems that are critical for life. We must consider our biological role as a part of these systems and think about how to be in harmony with it all. Most of us come from a culture that values domesticating our landscapes, and therefore we often feel a need to try to control the way nature works. We must give up the idea that our role is to own land and control it. In our time here on earth, we must create partnerships with the natural systems that support us, and we must also act as stewards for future generations by repairing ecological damage that has already been done and making decisions that will support the health of ecosystems long after we are gone.

Design of a sanctuary garden can be grounded in the same ethical guidelines that form the foundation of permaculture, a design approach to living sustainably on the earth. This summary of permaculture ethics states the guidelines I find most helpful in designing sacred spaces. Note that whenever one ethic seems to be in conflict with another, the first ethic trumps the rest. Refer to these ethics whenever you need to make a choice or resolve a problem.

* Care for the earth. Being good stewards of the planet comes first when we are designing anything. Creating spaces where well-being is the focus, we have a vested interest in maintaining functional ecosystems for our own health and prosperity. This means protecting ecosystem health and regenerating or repairing degraded landscapes. It also means being careful about how much we consume in building our special sanctuary.

* Care for people. The space we design should also meet the needs of the people who will use it, as well as future generations. When our needs are met, we quickly realize the importance of being good stewards of the space that fulfills these needs. We also understand that it's worth planting trees that won't produce a harvest in our lifetime but will provide sanctuary for those yet unborn.

* Give back. We need to share the abundance and surplus of the yields we enjoy from our sanctuary. When we feel improved well-being as a result of finding everyday sanctuary, we want to reinvest this in caring for the earth and people. This could mean that we share our resources, be it extra time, food, or money, to serve the first two ethics.

* Pace yourself. It's not just about the end goal but also about how we get there. The approach we use is just as important as the end product. We want to acknowledge that any transition takes time. We are not going to change overnight from stressed-out urban dwellers to perfectly balanced beings who incorporate nature's gifts into our daily routines. We must be

patient with ourselves as we engage the question of how to find everyday sanctuary and as we form new, healthier habits in our lives. Building our sanctuary space and practices may take a period of years and is best understood as an ongoing journey toward wellness.

Getting to Know the Spirit of the Land

All land has a history, rich with the footprints of many ancestors who once walked it; all land is full of life with species that often have symbiotic relationships; and all land has a unique energetic personality or *spiritus mundi*. Land inherently wants to be wild; as we ask it to meet our needs, we must respect it and seek a harmonious balance. If we listen to the land, it can help teach us what it wants to become and guide us in shaping it into a sanctuary. Reading books and taking classes, though useful, can only take us so far. We must open our minds and hearts to the spirit of the land to know what is possible.

As you begin to create a sacred space of your own, your respect for the land—and therefore for all land—will grow, and you will start to be able to discern healthy places from unhealthy places almost intuitively. To start off in a positive way, tune in to the spirit of the area you are thinking of carving out as sacred, whether it be a postage stamp of land in the city, a quarter-acre lot in the suburbs, or multiple acres in the countryside. Deeply experiencing the present reality of your space is your starting point. From here, you can begin to envision what could be.

Getting to know the land also involves observing these basic aspects of its ecosystem:

* Soil: What is its condition? Is it more clay, loam, or sand? Is it compacted or fluffy and full of organic matter? Which areas remain soggy after a rainfall and which areas drain quickly?

* Water: What are the sources of water on the land? Where does the water go when it runs off the roof and paving during a rainstorm?

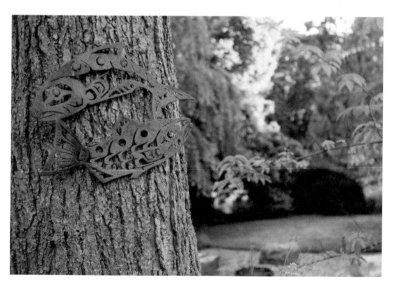

Indigenous salmon art pays respect to the Native American ancestors who walked so delicately on the earth.

MEDITATION
MEET THE GARDEN SPIRIT

Give yourself a minimum of five minutes to do this or take
as long as you like.

·1·

Sitting comfortably in your green space, close
your eyes and breathe deeply into your belly.

·2·

After ten or so deep breaths, open your eyes and ask
that the spirit of the land be with you. Ask it to offer
you assistance in learning about what it has the potential to become and how it can offer you sanctuary.

·3·

Experience the land with every sense, and take mental
note of all you notice. Feel the breeze on your skin, the
soil under your feet, the temperature. Smell and taste the
air and the fragrance of any plants around you. Listen to
the wind, the animals and insects nearby—as well as any
cars or other sounds of human presence. Look around.

·4·

See if you notice any differences from when you first
sat down. Do any specific areas of the land seem
to be trying to draw your attention to them?

·5·

Write down your observations and record your experiences.

* Flora and fauna: Which herbs, shrubs, vines, trees, and weeds are already growing in the space? Which creatures are regular visitors?

* Sun and shade: As the sun shifts in the sky during the procession of the seasons, which areas are shaded and which are in full sun? Where do you need more shade, where would you like more sun, and how can you maximize your use of the sun you do get?

To help yourself start envisioning the design of your sacred space, create a drawing of the land as it is. This could be as simple as a sketch by hand or a print-out of a satellite image from the Internet. Include the structural elements that are staying in place—rooflines, trees and drip lines, driveways and hardscape such as sidewalks, patios, raised beds, and arbors. Make several copies to draw on.

Then work through each aspect of the ecosystem in its current state, not-ing what needs help or healing. Track and make note of where the water runs through the space, where the soil is rich and where it is depleted, where it is wet or dry. Note where the existing plants are. Look at your land with beginner's eyes by sitting in multiple places at different times of day and noticing vistas. Lie on the ground. Stand right up against the fence to get the broadest view possible. Note views on your drawing. You can design the space to emphasize appealing vistas, whether a view of the sunset, natural features, or an artful object or area. Whatever you do, you will want to feel as if you are cooperating with the spirit of the land. We will return to working on your drawing later in this chapter.

Setting Specific Intentions

Too often we see gardens created simply to "landscape" an area. That effort may result in something pretty, but it will be devoid of deeper meaning. Typically a new home or building is constructed only with the intention of appealing to the widest possible range of buyers! Developers are infamous for cutting corners and especially for skipping important ecological design steps like considering soil or choosing plants that will grow to maturity without needing a constant haircut. They will often buy the least expensive plant available if it looks nice at the moment, not thinking ahead. Sometimes a garden will go through several owners before finding someone who truly loves it and wants to have a relationship with the space. By then, the plants are often tired from being mistreated and are barely hanging on with doses of fertilizer and timed irrigation, which act as life support.

In contrast, sacred spaces around the world share a common theme: they are always associated with a very specific intention. The next important step in creating sacred space for yourself is to define how you hope to use it. Think about your end goals, the aim of your desires and what you wish you could add space for in your life. For some people, it may simply be a quiet place that they can come home to, relax in, and find peace in after a long day at work. Some spaces may be devoted to prayer or even just to daydreaming. You can create a garden that heals—your body, mind, and soul. You can also create a space with different quadrants devoted to different intentions. For many people with limited space, one garden will have to serve multiple family needs. Perhaps you'd like a family gathering fire pit area and also an altar where you can honor your ancestors.

These are some common intentions for sacred spaces:

* prayer
* healing
* worship
* meditation
* performing rituals and ceremonies
* practicing yoga or qigong
* growing medicine
* boosting energy
* rejuvenation
* relaxation

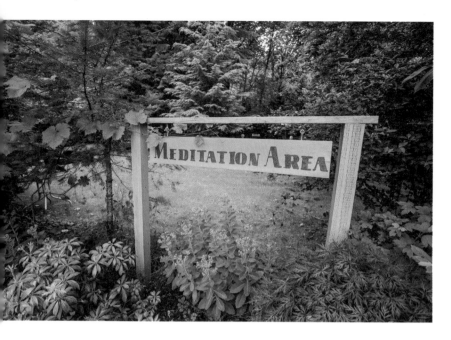

Signage for sacred spaces helps define intentions for users.

* burial/memorializing

* purification

* amplifying emotions

* enhancing creativity

* cleansing

When you have formulated your intentions, write them down. Keep them in front of you as you go through the process of fully imagining your green sanctuary and creating a list of desired features.

Finding Sources of Inspiration

Once you have tuned in to the spirit of the land and started to think about your intentions, there are a few more things you can do to aid the dreaming process. One is to gather ideas and be inspired by what others have done. When you can see the possibilities illustrated in concrete form, the creative juices flow more freely and you are more apt to move forward in fleshing out your dreams.

You might start by creating a "look book" in your notebook, journal, or binder with clippings and photographs. Consult sites such as Pinterest and Houzz to develop an idea board online. Go on garden tours and visit botanical gardens or nature preserves to find inspiration and see what types of plants and green spaces resonate with you. Places where plants have been nurtured and cared for well into maturity allow you to experience specimen trees, shrubs, and other flora in their full glory.

You can also visit sacred sites that are open to the public. There are thousands of such sites around the globe. Many are places where people over time have had noteworthy experiences or felt frequency differences in energy levels. Geological wonders, traditional places of pilgrimage or devotion, and historical sites all come to mind. Perhaps the best known of sacred spaces is Stonehenge in Wiltshire, England. It dates to at least 3000 BC, and its standing stones are positioned to align with significant seasonal events, such as sunrise on the summer solstice and sunset on the winter solstice. It was also

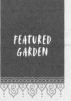

THE GARDEN *of* ANGELS

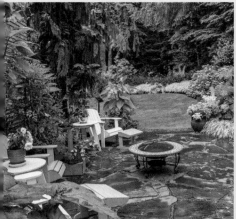
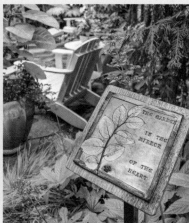
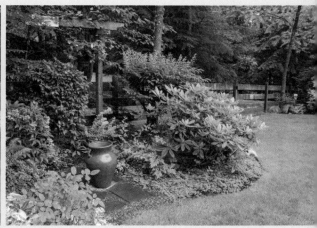

ABOVE, FROM LEFT TO RIGHT

The Petroviches' sanctuary includes a gathering area for family and friends.

Soulful signage reminds sanctuary visitors that tending the garden is also tending the heart.

A space was created with the intention of honoring Larry's father.

LARRY AND JANET PETROVICH live at the end of a long road deep in Snohomish County, Washington. Their idea of creating sanctuary began in 1997 with a newly purchased home and lots of lawn surrounded by a lush forest. Over the years, they have transformed their blank slate landscape into living spaces adorned with colorful art, meaningful memorials, and fun details. The plant life is diverse, with interesting textures and a playful ambiance. Tucked into the forest are walking trails and small garden spaces with dedications. A gravesite for an old pup is lovingly tended to and overlooked by an angel statue.

The two have created garden areas for their parents who have passed on and shared a love of gardening. Plants were chosen for sentimental reasons—"Mom

and Dad loved dogwoods. I always remember having one." Spending time in each garden helps them feel a connection to these beloved mentors. They plan to add cutting flowers that their parents loved as well so that they can bring these reminders inside their home. "There is no other place I'd rather be than digging in the dirt, being totally at peace in the garden—where God has blessed us with our own little piece of heaven on earth!"

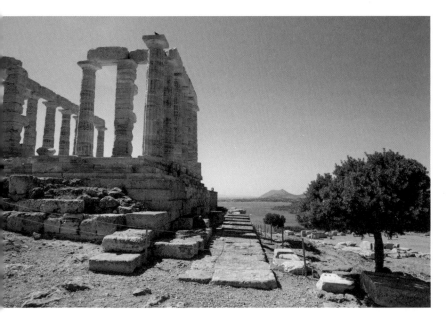

In the Mediterranean region, sacred spaces include ancient temples dating back to the fifth century BC. Pictured here, a single olive tree—among the most sacred plants in Greek mythology—stands next to the Temple of Poseidon near Athens.

BELOW Enchanted Rock State Natural Area in Texas features vernal pools and ghost footsteps, inspiration for combining stone and water in a sanctuary at home.

BELOW LEFT The Seven Sacred Pools in Sedona, Arizona, is another sacred site where water and stone combine.

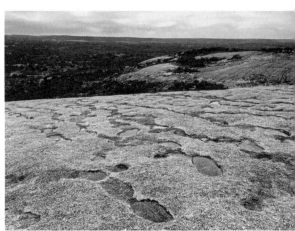

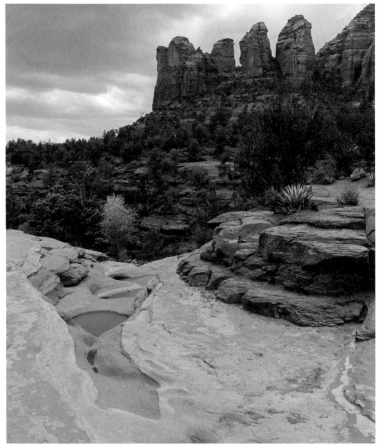

an important burial site. It was built with a specific intention and that intention has been respected, so it has retained significant spiritual and historical value.

In the United States, one renowned sacred place is Enchanted Rock, a massive pink granite dome in the Texas Hill Country that has been used for twelve thousand years as a ceremonial site. In addition to vernal pools and delicate ecosystems, it features "footsteps" imprinted in the rock, which legend says are the footsteps of ghosts who climb the rock every day—just one of many myths associated with the site.

Imagining with All Your Senses

Another thing you can do to aid the process of envisioning your sanctuary is to imagine how it will appeal to the various senses. We spend so much of our lives using just one or two senses—maybe squinting at a computer screen or gluing our ear to a phone—that our sanctuary garden may offer the best chance we have to enjoy the full spectrum of sensory pleasures. There we can stuff our eyes with color and texture, treat ourselves to soothing sound and stimulating scent, please our palates with sweet fruits and wholesome vegetables and nuts and herbs, trail our fingers in the water and shuffle our bare feet in the grass. All of these possibilities can be added to your list of desired features.

BELOW The palette of hot and cool colors in this container draws the eye in a celebration of late summer.

BELOW RIGHT This colorful array of flowers feels cheerful and wild.

COLOR AND TEXTURE

Using specific colors in your sanctuary is a way to evoke different emotions you may want to experience when you are in the space. What are your favorite colors? What moods do these evoke, and what feelings do they bring up? You can choose plants with these colors in their bark, flowers, or foliage, or you can add other colorful elements such as containers and painted walls, to help yourself feel a certain way in the garden. You can use masses of the same color in any area or create a wild mixture of colors.

Experiment with noticing how you feel in the presence of various colors. Cool colors such as green, blue, and violet tend to be calming, while hot colors such as reds and bright oranges can be energizing. You may instinctively know which colors

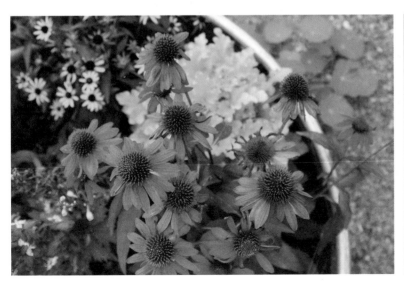

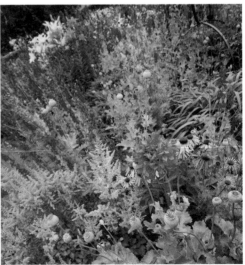

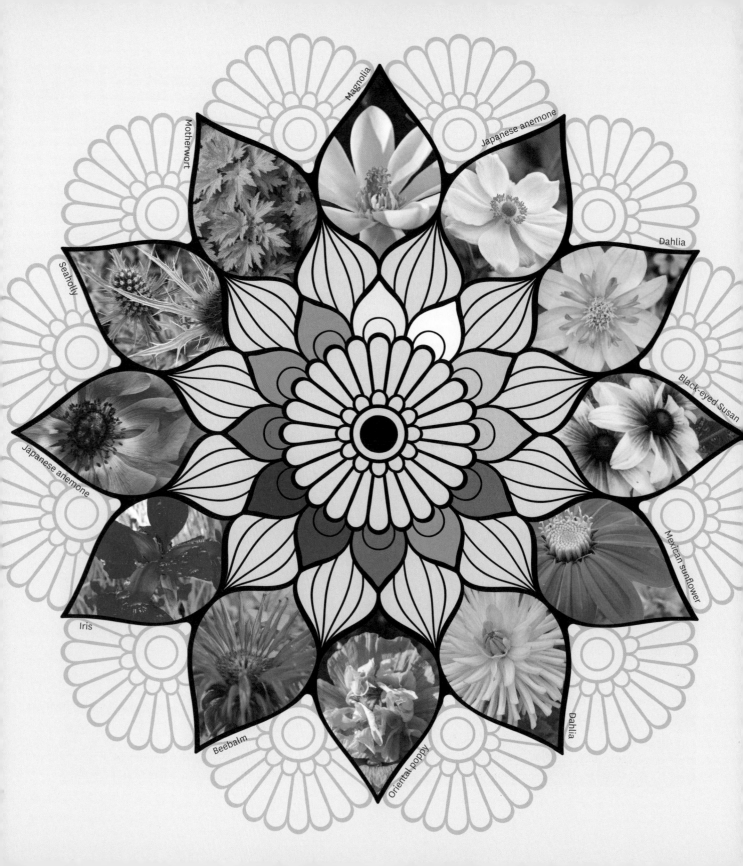

attract you and which repel you, which you want to include and which you want to avoid. The ancient Chinese practice of feng shui makes specific recommendations about where to place certain colors in relationship to the entrance and other energy centers in the garden. You can follow a formal system like this or trust your own intuition to guide you, which is my own preference. You might add more of the colors that represent qualities you want to increase in yourself or your life. Cool, calming colors can strengthen an inward spiritual focus, while warmer colors can help you feel vibrant and celebratory.

- white—purity, cleanliness, hope, freshness, modern feeling

- yellow—joy, fun, happiness, confidence

- orange—warmth, cheerfulness, creativity, fun, rejuvenation, optimism

- red—love, passion, vitality, power, anger, excitement, boldness, energy

- pink—romance, compassion, love, serenity, femininity

- purple—wisdom, creativity, luxury, quietude, reflection, royalty, dignity, magic, vision, spirituality

- blue—trust, strength, peace, tranquility, integrity, intelligence, coolness

- green—peace, growth, healing, safety, relaxation, balance, freshness

- brown—earthiness, authenticity, richness, simplicity, tradition

- black—sophistication, mystery, death, formality

- gray—calmness, stability, maturity, strength

Textural contrasts are also interesting and stimulating to eyes, especially to those that have stared at screens for too long. Every plant has its own unique aesthetic defined by overall form, size and shape of leaves, vein pattern, and presence of blossoms or berries. It's fun to pair one plant with another, or several, to make a beautiful tapestry in the garden. For example, the bold giant leaves of rhubarb or hosta play nicely with the smaller-cut leaves of ferns and creeping sedums. You can create patterns of these textural contrasts and repeat them throughout the garden. These rich layers of texture can set the mood of your sanctuary space—soft and subdued or bold and dramatic.

You can also add textures that are pleasant to touch, such as the soft leaves of lamb's ears, a cool spongy cushion of moss, or scented geraniums that reward your caress with a fuzzy texture and a whiff of relaxing fragrance.

SOOTHING SOUND

Noise pollution pervades our world and has a jarring effect on our nervous

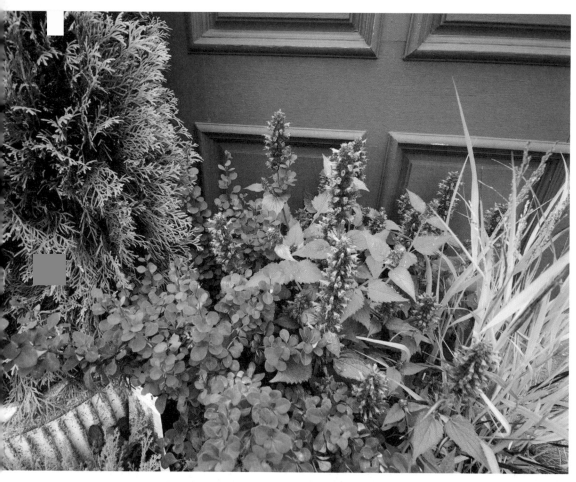

Combining false cypress, reddish Japanese barberry, hyssop, and a yellow grass with a purple door as backdrop is bold and fun.

BELOW LEFT The shapes of fern fronds and grasses contrast nicely with the backdrop of a large fir tree.

BELOW CENTER An interesting depth and contrast are created by the varying leaf sizes and patterns of hostas, Solomon's seal, and oxalis, plus the height of the container.

BELOW The bark of trees like this paper birch can add texture accents as well.

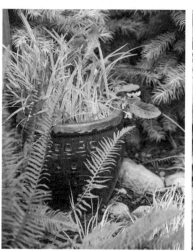

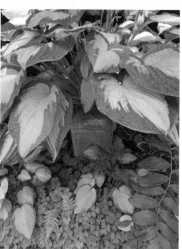

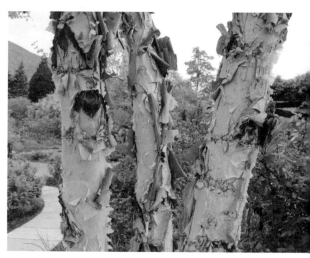

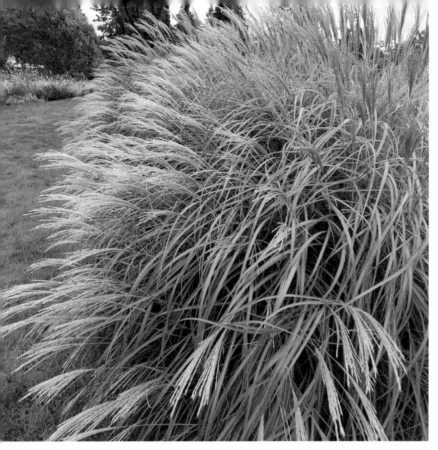

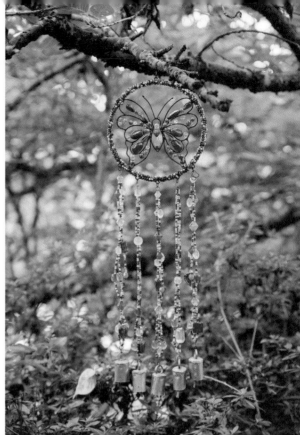

The sound of a summer breeze through miscanthus leaves can be mesmerizing.

ABOVE RIGHT These wind chimes serve as a piece of art and also provide a tinkling sound when played on by a current of air.

systems. The constant whizz of traffic, the clunk and screech of heavy machinery, the deafening squeal of a cappuccino machine, the artificial beeps and bleeps of electronic devices—these are everyday stressors most of us live with. Our ears crave the restful sounds of wind, water, and birdsong, and these can be part of any sanctuary garden, no matter how small.

Imagine the musical rustle of wind moving through aspen, cottonwood, eucalyptus, or bamboo leaves. Large grasses, seedpods, and wind chimes are also played upon by the wind. The sound of rain is peaceful and is amplified by a rain chain, which is a way to celebrate rainfall and create a gentle sound during a drizzle or music during a storm. Running water in fountains small or large or in watercourses that fill during a downpour can soothe our souls and refresh our ears, as well as providing drinking water to many creatures. The drowsy hum of insect voices on a summer afternoon can lull us into a meditative state.

FRAGRANCE

The sweet scent of star jasmine, honeysuckle, or Asiatic lilies on a warm summer

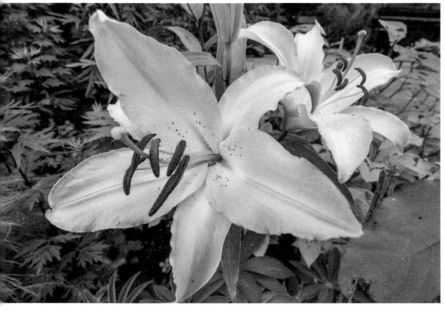

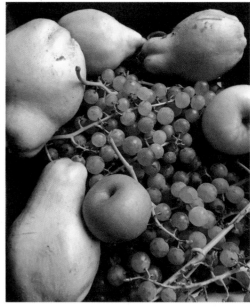

Asiatic lilies make great cut flowers and fill your garden with fragrance.

ABOVE RIGHT Fruit collected from the garden on a September afternoon includes grapes as well as Asian and European pears.

evening can add to the sense of being surrounded and protected in a sanctuary garden. Roses in bloom remind us to pause and breathe in, a welcome cue to slow down. What fragrance do you love that you could add to your personal Eden? You might want to envision paths and seating areas that bring you close to fragrant blossoms or put you in the way of wafting scents.

TASTE

What's more delicious than a perfectly red, ripe strawberry plucked and savored on an early June morning, or a raspberry eaten straight off the cane in midsummer? Edibles are an important element to consider adding to your sanctuary.

Berries are easy to grow in whatever space you have and add to the sense that your garden is a paradise on earth. Think of the pleasure of dashing out into the garden on a wintry afternoon to grab a handful of rosemary to toss with the potatoes roasting in the oven or to add to a pot of soup simmering on the stove. Anyone can plant a culinary herb garden, even on a kitchen windowsill.

Growing tree fruits and nuts takes more space and patience but can add considerably to meeting your needs for tasty nourishment. Cherry tomatoes can be popped into your mouth while you're harvesting squash and green beans for dinner, just a few of the many possibilities for growing healthy foods in a backyard sanctuary of any size.

DREAMING OF YOUR PARADISE

Taking a journey in your imagination to tap into sensory experience can help you get clues about what your own ideal sanctuary may be.

1· Get comfortable (sitting or lying down), relax, and close your eyes. Focus on taking several deep breaths and continue breathing deeply throughout the journey.

2· Start by thinking of what the word *paradise* brings up in your mind's eye. What do you see? Colors, people, plants, animals, locations, elements?

3· What do you hear? Wind, birds, talking, singing, a body of water?

4· What do you smell? Food, fragrance, plants, the weather changing?

5· What do you feel on your skin? The warmth of the sun, a gentle rain, a cool breeze?

6· What do you taste? The sweetness of fruit, the pungency of herbs?

7· What does your heart feel? Happiness, grief, joy, indifference?

8· Now open your eyes and write down what came to you.

You may want to do this process several times before you are feeling ready to move forward. See if you can identify one or more immediate additions or changes you can make to your yard to bring it more in alignment with your vision.

◆

Children's Sanctuary

If you have children in your life, your everyday sanctuary can include a space for them. Children are precious, our future, our hope. Wendell Berry writes, "Teaching children about the natural world should be treated as one of the most important events in their lives." We should expose them to the outdoors and to life beyond themselves as much as possible, as this can bring about so many great opportunities for learning. Not only does outdoor play develop motor and sensory skills, but it can also teach compassion, patience, and acceptance. Outdoors, children can develop a relationship with other creatures, experiencing an empathetic connection they will most likely carry with them throughout life. Children's natural curiosity leads them on. My sons began collecting different types of rocks, and it eventually became a ritual on every family vacation to visit geological features and rock shops.

Do you remember the first plant you had a relationship with? Or the first animal you met that became a friend? Drawing on your own memories can help you imagine how to create a children's sanctuary. You might want to build an enchanted realm there. Although some adults may turn their noses up at the idea of magical beings residing in green areas, it especially resonates with children and those who

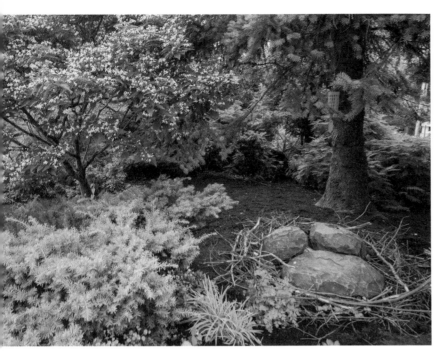

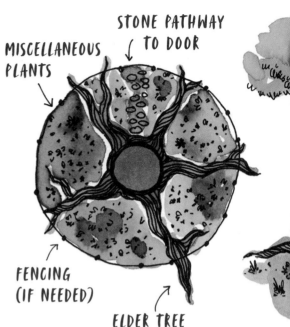

MISCELLANEOUS PLANTS

STONE PATHWAY TO DOOR

FENCING (IF NEEDED)

ELDER TREE

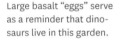

Large basalt "eggs" serve as a reminder that dinosaurs live in this garden.

believe in magic. Creating special sanctuaries for creatures such as fairies can catch the imagination and encourage children to spend time outdoors looking for them, creating natural "homes" for them, and learning an appreciation for the natural world in the process. For ages, these spirit allies, including elves, sprites, angels, nymphs, pixies, and goblins, have been called upon for help. So how do we create an environment to attract these mystical allies?

1 Hold good intentions—be kind, believe in them and welcome them.

2 Create a safe, dedicated space for them.

3 Incorporate an assortment of flowers, foliage, and fruit that you imagine they can use.

4 Include colorful objects such as flags and ornaments that you think might appeal to small beings.

5 Add wind chimes or other items that make sounds to call the fairy beings in.

Charting and Sketching Your Plan

This chapter has given you a few ways to begin envisioning your ideal sanctuary and has also encouraged you to think about how your own preferences might mesh with the spirit of the land. At this point a good way to crystallize your impressions is to make a simple chart listing your needs, wants, and desires. Needs are what you cannot live without. Wants are the elements you'd like to have but can live without. Desires are the elements that would be nice to have but are lower priority than wants and can be added later. Ultimately you are looking for what will make you feel fully restored and help you live in harmony with the earth.

Here are some examples:

Needs	Wants	Desires
safety	children's garden	water features
privacy	chickens	meditation space
food	rain collection	composting
medicine		

Remember: take care of the earth, and the earth will take care of you. As you carefully consider what you need, want, and desire, think about what the land can offer and how you can support the land in providing this sustainably. For example, if one of the intentions of your sanctuary is to grow food and medicine, you will need to support the land in providing the necessary soil, water, and sunlight. We will return to the needs of the land in the chapter "Five Steps to Creating Your Sanctuary Garden."

Now take out the sketch you did of your land and note where you might situate each of your needed, wanted, and desired features. For example, a grassy area in full sun is a perfect space for a vegetable garden; the shaded area under a large old tree might be used to shelter a quiet meditation bench.

All sacred spaces we create should evoke a sense of harmony and peace when we enter and use them. We must consider the natural ecological function of the space and make sure that the space can support our goals to use it for ourselves. This is where the ethical guidelines outlined at the beginning of the chapter come in. As you reflect on the various aspects of what you envision for your sacred space, ask yourself: Are my choices good for the earth? Are they good for the people? Will these choices be ecologically regenerative and implemented in a process I can manage—physically, financially, emotionally? Evaluate your plan and reassess until you feel comfortable moving forward.

The next chapter will give you some ideas and examples of elements you might want to include in your sanctuary to help you realize your intention or intentions and fulfill your needs, wants, and desires for the area.

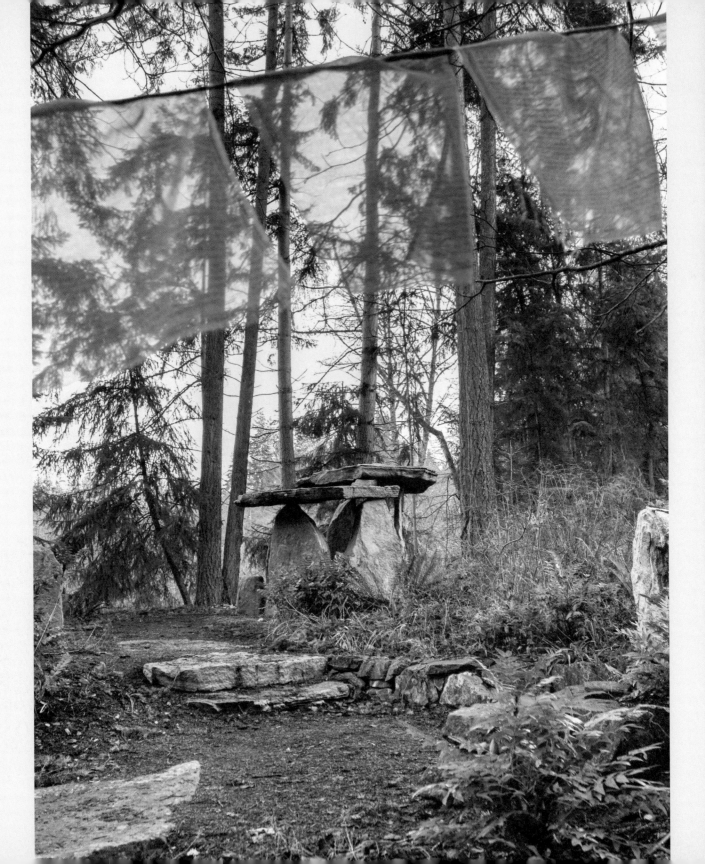

Common Elements of Sacred Spaces

Prayer flags hang over standing stones at Earth Sanctuary on Whidbey Island, Washington.

RIGHT Gates come in a wide range of styles, but all act as portals into a space with specific uses.

When you have a clear intention for and vision of your sacred space, you can go about filling it with resources to support your vision. Sacred spaces contain different elements depending on the intent of the space and goals of its creator, but the elements described and shown in this chapter are often found in many of them. These are also things that can easily be incorporated into a garden. Add images or a list of any of these that appeal to you to your notebook, journal, or binder of ideas.

The Threshold, Portal, or Entrance

A good way to announce a sacred space—and to remind yourself to be reverent every time you enter—is some kind of demarcation that lets visitors know they are entering into a special area with specific uses. Arches or gates to pass through give the user an experience of physical transition and can often lead to a more grounded or meaningful experience. Some sacred spaces have signs posted outside of their gates that let visitors know any rules to follow. You should feel free to create some of your own or to post a meaningful quote or the name of the space on a placard.

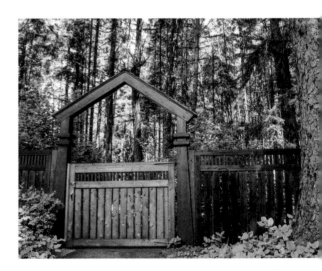

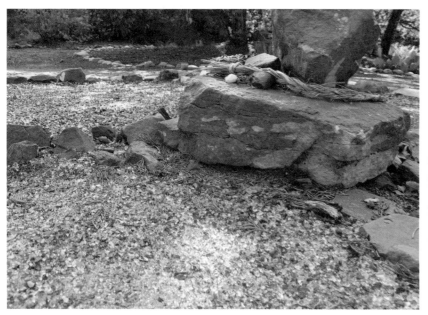

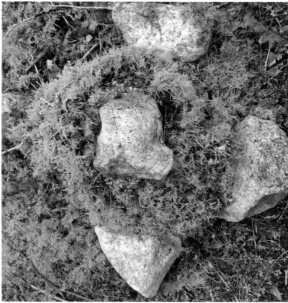

Altars can be placed atop logs or stones to raise them up off the ground.

ABOVE RIGHT This small stone altar marks south in a ceremonial space.

Altars

If you visit any church or religious space, you are likely to see an altar or two … or more. People have been creating altars for thousands of years for both personal use and larger community purposes. Altars hold an intention or focus energy toward some goal such as assisting transformation, honoring or remembering a person or place, or creating community. They can be used for healing, to recharge energy, or for any other specific purpose.

Altars can be created in any indoor or outdoor space. Outdoors, they can be placed atop stones or logs, anything that raises them up from the ground. Objects are placed on the altar to serve as reminders, to hold energy, or to serve the intention the altar was built for. These objects can be placed to mark the four cardinal directions. The altar can be changed after the original intention has been fulfilled or when a new intention takes shape.

Bells and Chimes

In a sacred space, the sounds of bells and chimes aid in awakening or changing the energy of those within earshot. Some tones are used to bless a space, while others are known to chase away evil spirits. The sounds produced and the frequencies at which they resonate depend on the material and form of the bell or chime. Those that resonate with deep, low

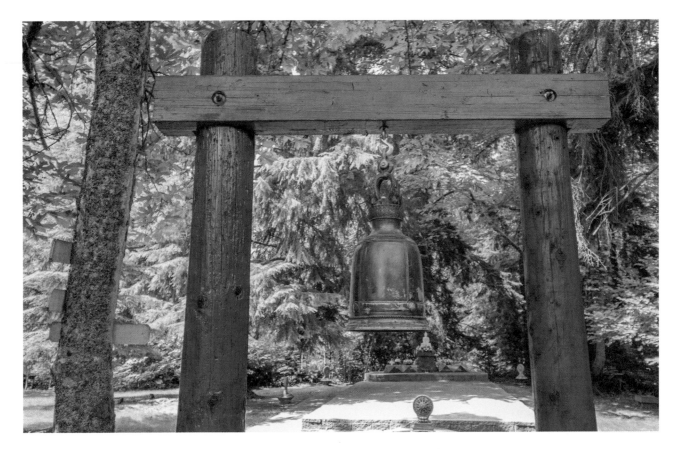

This bell is used in a ceremonial space at the Atammayatarama Buddhist Monastery in Woodinville, Washington.

RIGHT A bell hanging from a tree along a path at Earth Sanctuary can be rung by visitors or by the elements.

tones can often help us feel soothed and grounded. Others with higher tones can help us feel clearer and more alert.

Bells, chimes, and gongs can be rung at certain times of day to mark mealtimes or the beginnings and endings of prayer or meditation. Chimes can also give an added voice to natural elements like wind and rain. A soft breeze playing with chimes sounds completely different from a wild windstorm causing the chimes to clatter and bang against each other.

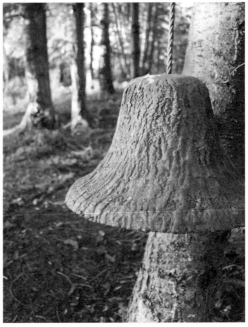

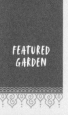

GHOSTHORSE HOLLOW

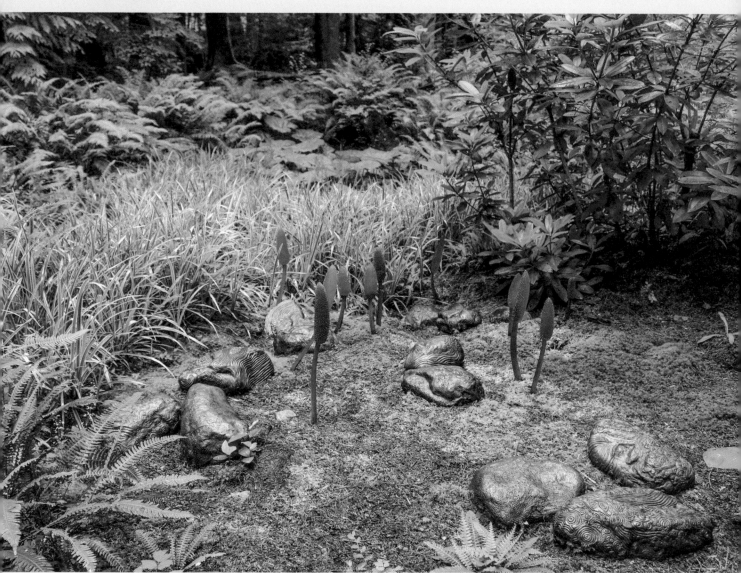

Flame pods made of acrylic
resin and dye glow in
late afternoon when the
setting sun hits them.

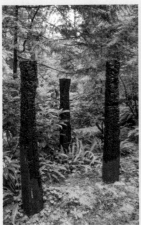 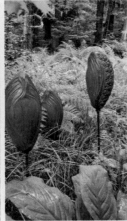 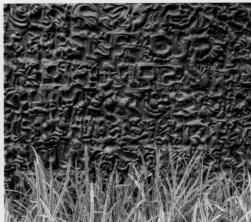 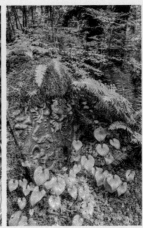

Charred pillars of painted wood stand tall amidst the native foliage.

These blue pods made of resin colored with automotive paint rise up from a sea of sedge and skunk cabbage.

The Earth Code wall is a retaining wall made of pigmented cement stained with acid.

The Rune Stones are large concrete tiles with a black powder-infused coating placed along the trails to add mystery, contrast, and rhythm.

DEEP IN A MOSSY FOREST near Monroe, Washington, lies an enchanting sanctuary filled with whimsical biomorphic art. One of the most fascinating gardens I've ever visited, Ghosthorse Hollow is the home of graphic artist and sculptor Robert Fairfax and his wife, Nancy. The 5-acre site has a creek running through it, and Fairfax has honored the land by harmonizing his home and his art with the surrounding mixture of woods and wetlands. He has turned the meticulously nurtured ecological garden into an outdoor sculpture gallery, with trails meandering throughout that reveal art at each turn.

His art is made of all sorts of mediums, from resin to wood to metal. There are portals and entrances, a memorial to his mother made of undulating black concrete pillars that he calls the Spirit Arbor, and other functional features like walls and cube seats as well as standalone specimens. Burnt posts are striking landmarks rising up out of ferns and moss. Some of my favorite installations look like colonies of alien life forms emerging from the pockets of wetland ecosystems. Playful urchins and colorful pods peek out among native sedge and skunk cabbage as if they were newly emerging species. The land vibrates with life and magic.

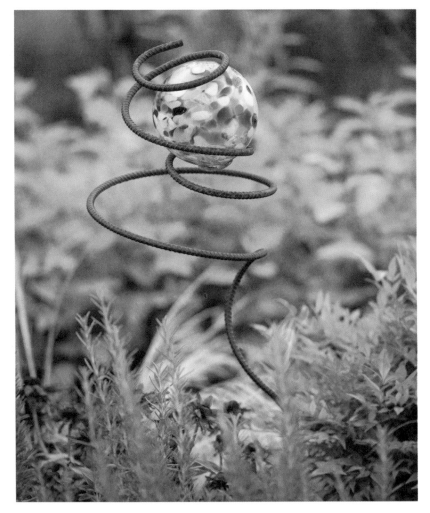

Garden Art

Art can add soulful expression to a sacred space and can complement earth elements like plants and stones. Statues, sundials, large sculptures, and small ephemeral offerings of plants that are in bloom are among the almost endless possibilities. Art can serve as the main focal point in a sacred space and/or as a subtle reminder or message hidden in the foliage. When considering art, choose something that is personally meaningful and evokes emotions you want to feel. Ask how it will hold up in the weather if you want it to be permanent. And remember that less is more, as too much art in a space can lose its power and just seem overwhelming or cluttering.

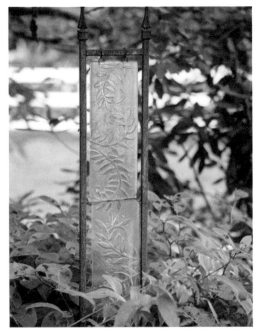

A colorful glass orb adds a touch of whimsy to the garden—especially in winter when many of the plants are dormant.

RIGHT This unique art came from a grandfather's playful game of hiding for his grandchildren all the letters that spell their last name; this is the letter o.

FAR RIGHT As the natural light changes throughout the day, this etched glass piece takes on different appearances.

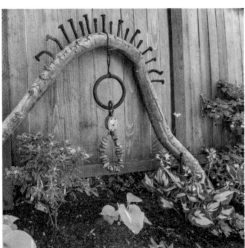

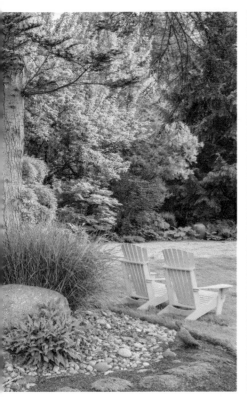

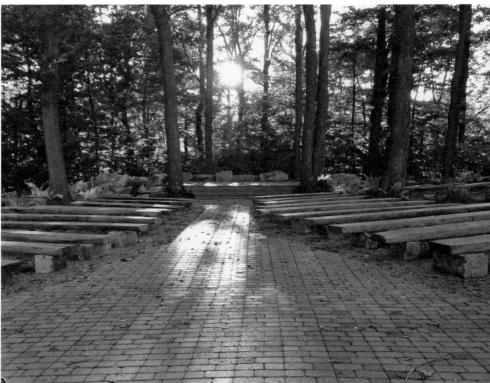

Well-placed chairs can encourage two or more people to gather and visit.

ABOVE RIGHT This seating arrangement is for large gatherings such as ceremonies, performances, and celebrations.

Gathering Places

Sacred spaces often feature gathering places for social interaction that are safe and welcoming. Some may be for prayer or ceremony, some for festivities and celebration. Think of sweat lodges as an example of the first type and maypoles as an illustration of the second. Some are on an intimate scale and others are large enough for community events. Ideally, a gathering place should have some flexibility as far as the kinds of activities that can happen there as well as the amenities it offers, such as seating or a stage area for performances. Simple and inexpensive seating can include log rounds, rocks, or salvaged lumber propped up on cement blocks. If a gathering place is going to serve many people, it is best created in collaboration to reflect the needs and culture of those who will be using it.

FIRE PITS

Fire is a powerful transformative element in nature, and the comfort of gathering around a small fire to find warmth, to cook, to tell stories, and to enact rituals is engrained in our species memory. Fire

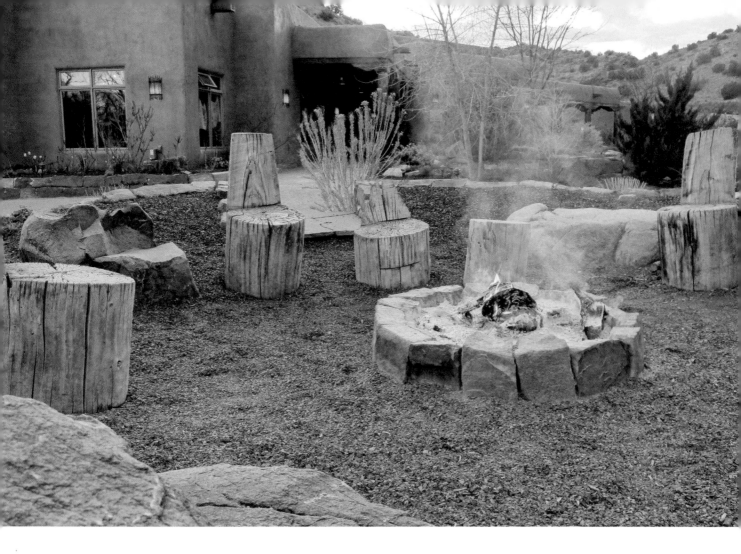

This fire pit at Ojo Caliente Mineral Springs in New Mexico is made from local stone and serves as a central gathering place for guests when they are not using the healing mineral pools.

pits or circles can be simple or elaborate. The simplest consist of a hole dug in the ground lined with rocks. Fire containers manufactured from metal, terra cotta, or stone come in all shapes, sizes, and costs. It is important to consider seating around the fire and how close people need to be to fully experience the fire's warmth. I often suggest using log rounds, which can easily be moved by rolling them, but for more permanence, stones add to the earthy ambience and won't

need to be replaced. Or leave it open to chairs that can be brought in and taken away. Another important consideration is ensuring that the ground and surroundings are fireproof in case an ember or spark flies out of the pit.

MEMORIALS

Memorials are gathering places for honoring our loved ones and ancestors, for celebrating lives once lived. A sacred

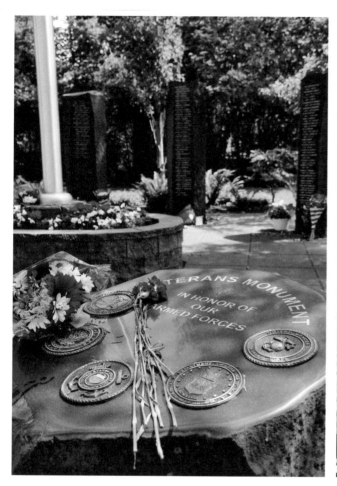

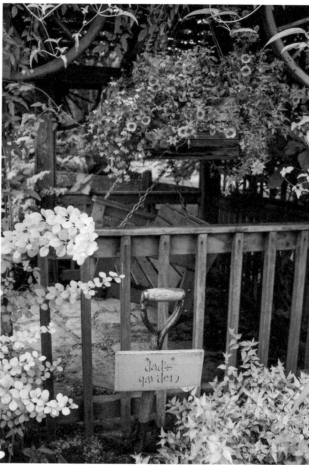

The Veterans Memorial Garden in Mill Creek, Washington, is a place where events and ceremonies honoring those who have served in the military take place several times a year.

ABOVE RIGHT A memorial garden for an individual can include plants that were special to that person.

space can be created solely for memorial purposes, or part of a sacred space can be devoted to elements and objects that are sentimental and hold memories. Using plants loved by departed ones is a way to make it a place that carries their spirit well after they are gone, a place to visit and find solace. Memorials can also include burial grounds, such as places where pets are laid to rest.

Lanterns/Light

Sacred spaces often use natural or installed lighting to create a desired effect. Throughout the seasons as the sun and moon move through the sky, they have different illuminating effects. Closer to the summer equinox, the sun is out for a longer period and moves through the sky on a higher trajectory than during the winter months, when it travels lower on the horizon and is present for fewer hours.

Objects can be placed intentionally to catch light at certain times of the year. For instance, in a memorial garden celebrating an ancestor's birthday, an altar or focal area can be placed where the sun will fall directly upon it on that day.

With installed lighting, less is more. Using downlights or uplighting an object or tree can create dramatic effects, but artificial light in the dark also attracts night creatures such as moths and bats

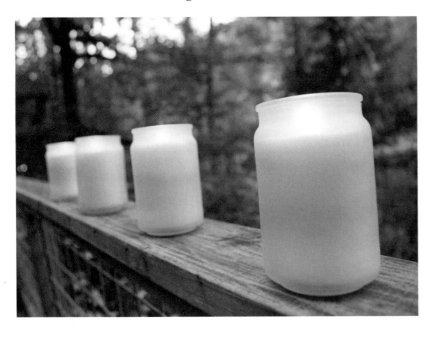

Candles can create a warm ambience in your sanctuary space.

and can create light pollution. Lanterns or lit candles in carriers can be a good choice to illuminate special occasions, as long as safety precautions are observed. If you want to use string lights on a plant, be careful not to attach the string too tightly and do not leave the lights on any longer than necessary.

Mandalas

A mandala is a universal pattern that has found expression in many different cultures across time. *Mandala* translates to "circle" in Sanskrit, but mandalas can be square as well. The pattern inside of the circle or square is concentric—organized around a unifying center. The mandala pattern has special significance in Eastern religions, used as a focus of meditation, but it is also found in expressions such as labyrinths and medicine wheels. Both Tibetan monks and Navajo Indians create elaborate sand mandalas to demonstrate the reality of impermanence. Mandalas are used in sacred spaces as a template for laying out beds and paths and also as works of art.

LABYRINTHS

Labyrinths, a form of mandala dating back to prehistoric times, have been built around the world, at churches, in parks, and in backyards, with many different purposes in mind, including trapping spirits and representing the path to God. While a maze goes off in many directions and is meant to confuse or cause the walker to get lost, a labyrinth's path guides the walker to one central spot. Modern labyrinths are usually walked in a meditative or prayerful state, often symbolizing the act of going within ourselves. We can walk them for a specific healing

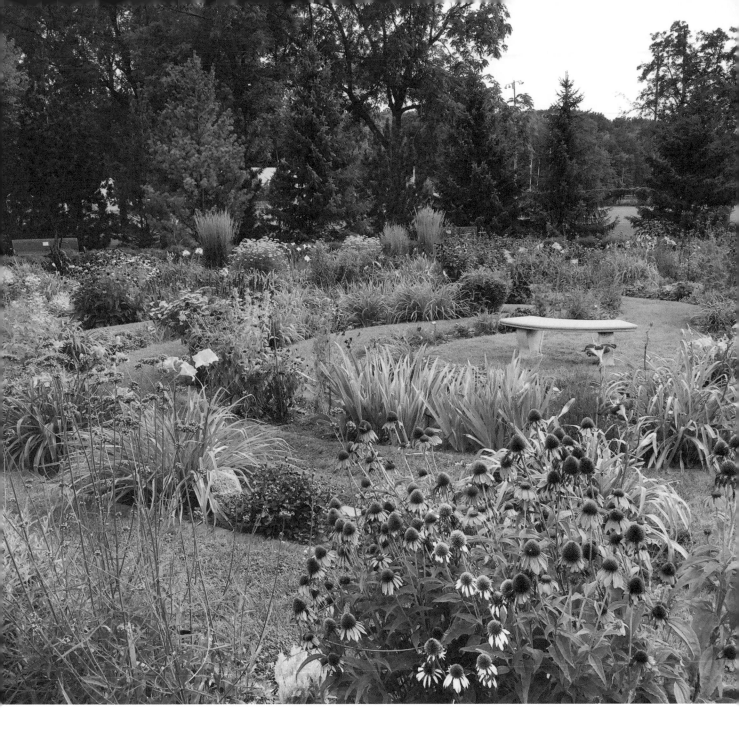

The colorful Labyrinth Garden Earth Sculpture in a park in West Bend, Wisconsin, is a design from Crete created and maintained by the community.

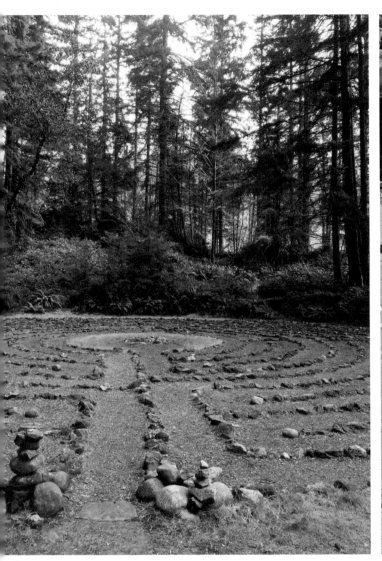

A labyrinth at the Whidbey Institute, a center for transformative learning in Clinton, Washington, is laid out in a classical pattern.

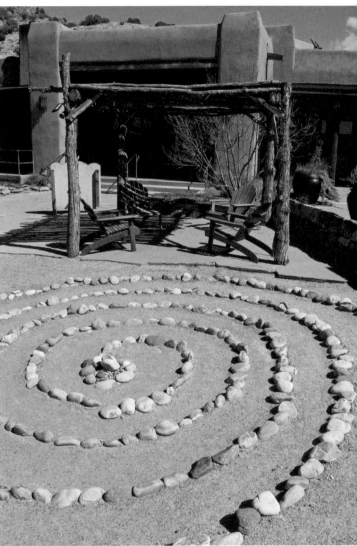

A spiral labyrinth invites guests at the Ojo Caliente hot springs resort to take a meditative walk toward their inner selves.

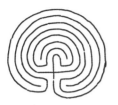 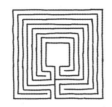 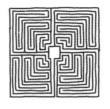 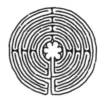 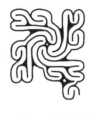

CLASSICAL   ROMAN   MEDIEVAL   CONTEMPORARY

Labyrinth patterns and
shapes, from classi-
cal to contemporary

Sacred geometry

If you look around, you will see that sacred geometry exists all over our world. Sacred geometry tells us that certain geometric shapes and proportions have symbolic meanings that are sacred. This belief system also suggests that all material forms are expressions of an underlying geometry.

Shapes such as circles, spirals, and hexagons were used in the architecture of ancient sacred structures and are used today in the design of religious buildings such as churches, temples, and mosques. These same patterns are also found in nature—in seeds, flowers, shells, honeycombs, leaves, in the eye of a storm. We can design spaces or art to use simple geometric shapes as well as more complex shapes such as fractals and branching patterns. These patterns can be appreciated for their beauty and their symbolic meanings, and they can also result in designs that make efficient and resilient use of energy and space.

purpose, to pray for help or guidance, to connect to spirit, or simply to find solace and clarity.

Labyrinths can be elaborate or simple. They can be laid out in a variety of patterns and shapes, and made from a variety of materials. Stones can be laid on top of the soil, pavers can be cut into sod, edges can be outlined with paint or plants. Spiral labyrinths are particularly easy to lay out, and they echo patterns seen in natural objects such as seashells and natural events such as fern fronds unfolding.

MEDICINE WHEELS

In indigenous cultures around the world, the medicine wheel, or sacred hoop, pattern has been used in the landscape for

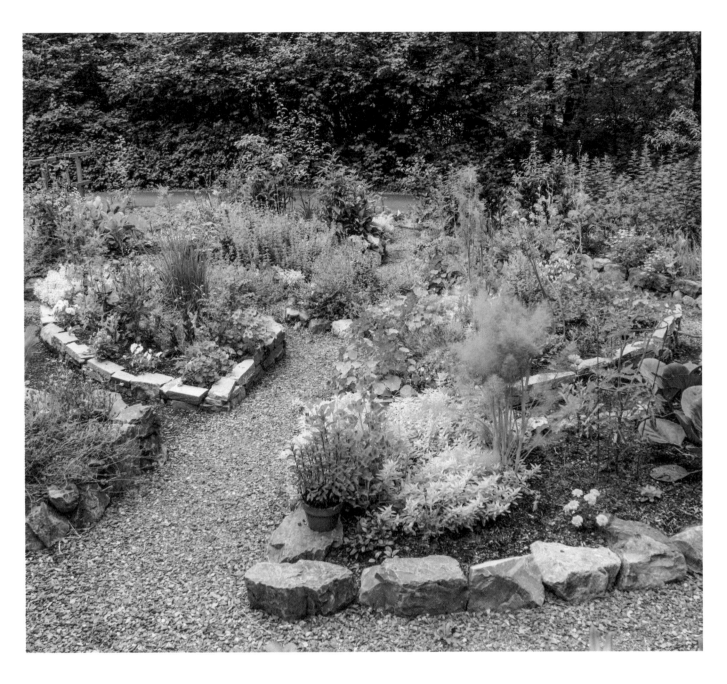

A healing garden laid out
in a medicine wheel is
used for growing edible
and medicinal plants.

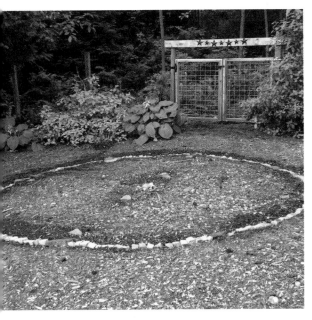

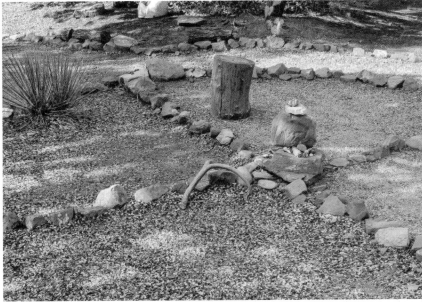

This simple medicine wheel garden has stones placed to mark the four directions.

ABOVE RIGHT A medicine wheel in Sedona, Arizona, has an altar at the center to provide a focal point for prayer and meditation.

thousands of years. The medicine wheel symbolizes the four directions and is a place of healing, harmony, community gathering, amplifying prayer, and connecting to spirit. The medicine wheel can take many forms but basically consists of a circle—usually made with stones—with a center and spokes radiating in the cardinal directions. Each direction is associated with a color, an earth element, a season, a time of day, a stage of life, or a type of plant or animal. The medicine wheel can be used as a format for many different kinds of teachings, and with the hundreds of lineages, each teaching is a little different.

Many gardeners and healers today are adopting the medicine wheel concept to create sacred space in their gardens. They gather materials that are significant to them and carefully place these materials to keep balance within the space. They position plants within the quadrants in a very intentional way. For instance, plants that bloom can be placed in the quadrant corresponding to the color of the flowers; herbs for treating ailments can be placed in the quadrant corresponding to the body part or condition to be treated. The circle can also contain cairns, an altar, offerings, and many more elements.

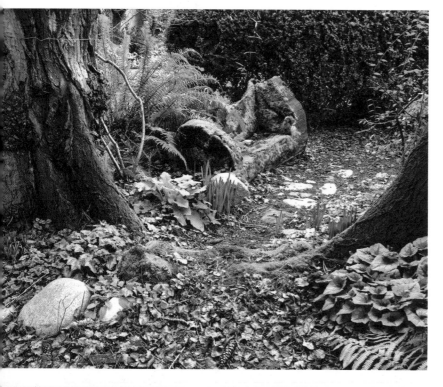

A rustic bench for one offers a quiet place for reflection and meditation protected by large trees.

BELOW This wishing tree in Seattle gathers the prayers of many individuals asking for help from the spirit of the tree.

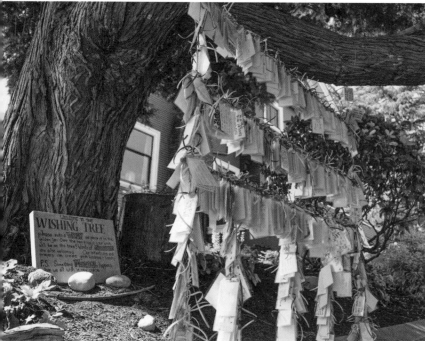

Prayer/Meditation and Yoga/Qigong Spaces

A powerful way to connect with the healing benefits of nature is to pray, meditate, and/or practice yoga or qigong outdoors. Sacred space can be planned to accommodate these uses. A peaceful deck or lawn can serve as a level place to do yoga poses and qigong movements. Prayer and meditation might take place in a protected corner or a quiet grove of trees with seating positioned for this purpose. Prayer flags can be inscribed with intentions or prayers and strung around the space in a tradition that began in Tibet more than two thousand years ago. Tibetans believe that when these flags flap in the breeze, they carry the prayers and blessings printed on them to the land and the community.

Stones

Stones are the keepers and holders of energy. Standing stones such as those at Stonehenge—either solitary or arranged in circles or rows—have been discovered at

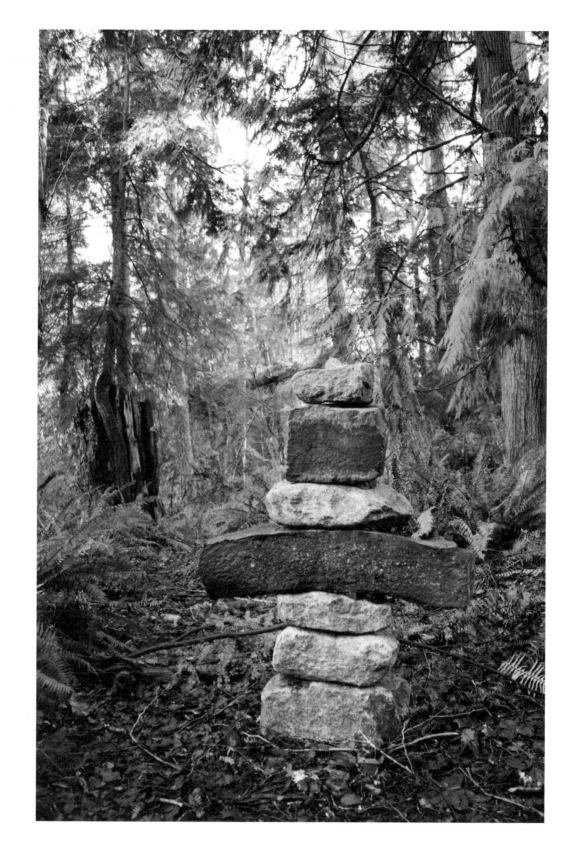

Cairns can be made in different sizes and shapes from different types of stones.

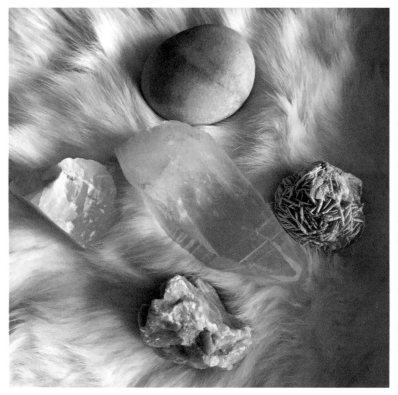

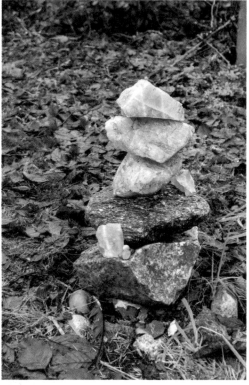

Stones and crystals come in all shapes, sizes, and colors, each carrying different energies.

ABOVE RIGHT Rose quartz, believed to open and purify the heart, is used in this small cairn.

sites around the world and were probably used in rituals and ceremonies and for astronomical observations. No one knows for certain how these stones were moved into place, since contemporary monoliths and stone circles are usually placed with heavy equipment.

Also found throughout the world but easier to assemble are stacks of stones called cairns. Cairns can be markers for burial sites, cues for trail navigation, pointers to astrological wonders, or reminders of specific geographical or historical information about a site. More modern cairns are often used in gardens as art or landscape markers. The process of building

them can facilitate prayers or meditation. I tell my clients that if they ask and listen, certain stones will talk to them and impart their wisdom, a practice that makes sense if you consider that most stones have been here far longer than humans.

Some cairns feature crystals, stones with unique properties that have been used for healing since ancient times. Crystals are understood to change the frequency of auras and absorb negative energies, and can be used as tools or sacred objects in the spaces we are creating. Different crystals have traditionally been associated with different applications, and the way they are used in a sacred space depends to some extent on the relationship to them cultivated by the person using them. Here are a few common types of crystals:

* agate: helps with balancing personal energy, healing, and cleansing

* amethyst: confers protection from negativity, sharpens intuition, and can be used to cleanse sacred space

* citrine: aids in manifesting, creating success, and attracting love and happiness

* moonstone: helps us go with the flow, aids emotional health, confers protection and good fortune

* obsidian: protects and grounds, helps to heal trauma and self-limiting beliefs

* quartz: provides healing energy and amplifies intentions and prayers

Water Features

Water is sacred; water is life. Having water as an element in a sacred space is a good idea if that land and its natural resources support it. Water is cleansing, can be soothing to the soul, and can symbolize emotion, clarity, and purity. A quiet pond can encourage reflection, while a bubbling creek provides soothing sounds and supports wildlife. Sometimes a water element is naturally occurring, and sometimes it is human made. I often include a small recirculating bubbling stone or a large water bowl or rain chain in the sacred spaces I design. Varying degrees of maintenance are needed, but these features can also be turned off or emptied if appropriate.

This fountain was designed to trickle droplets off of the plants growing at the top, to offer a subtle and tranquil ambiance.

FAR RIGHT A simple water feature adds beauty and sound and also offers an essential element for wildlife.

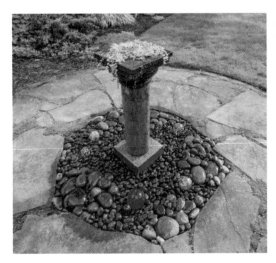

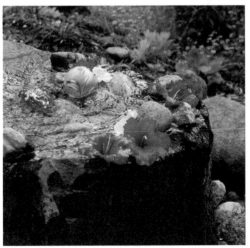

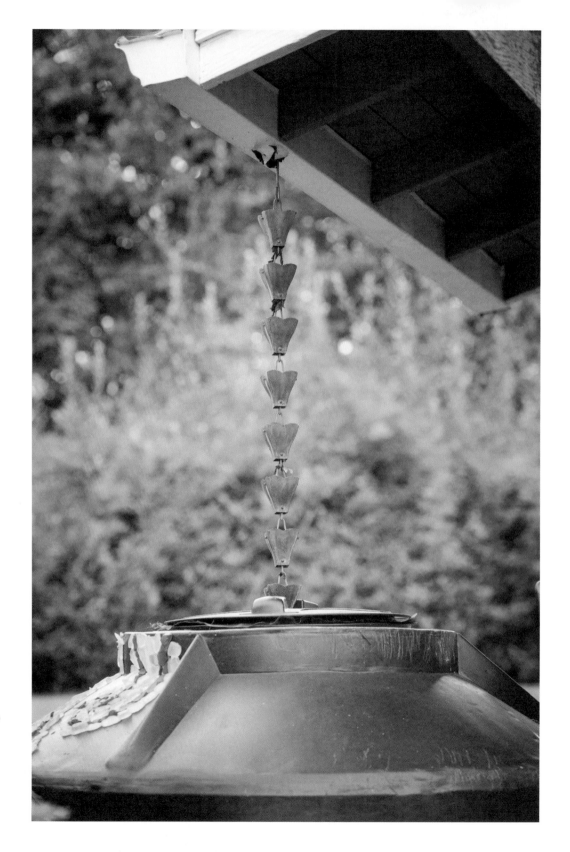

A rain chain is a way to celebrate rainfall and create a gentle sound during a drizzle or music during a storm.

EARTH SANCTUARY

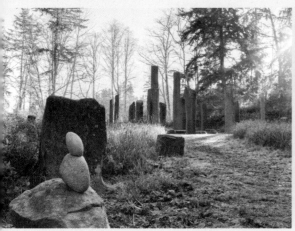
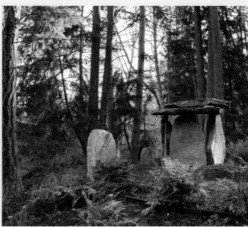
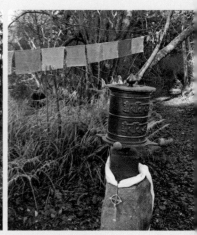

ABOVE, FROM LEFT TO RIGHT

A cairn sits at the entrance of a sacred space with monolithic columns in a circle.

Earth Sanctuary features a dolmen, a megalith of upright stones supporting a large horizontal slab.

Tibetan prayer flags and a prayer wheel release prayers into the wind at Earth Sanctuary.

CHUCK PETTIS, founder of Earth Sanctuary, a 72-acre nature preserve on Whidbey Island in Washington, is an expert on designing and creating sacred spaces as well as a successful business-man. With Earth Sanctuary, he undertook the task of restoring a piece of land that had been logged over in the early 1980s. His intention is to return the acreage to mature old-growth forest with a diversity of plant and animal life, and he has a five-hundred-year plan for doing this. In the meantime, the place offers an inspir-ing and unique environment for personal renewal and spiritual growth. Visitors come from all over to experience the many installations and spaces that honor diverse global spiritual traditions.

Perhaps most notable are two circles of standing stones—one 40 feet in diameter with stones 11 feet high, the other 16 feet in diameter with stones up to 7 feet high—that offer places for meditation and seasonal ceremony. Earth Sanctuary also features a dolmen, a mega-lith of upright stones supporting a large horizontal slab. Cairns of stacked stone grace the forest trails. A labyrinth made of Pennsylvania bluestone and outlined with native salal hedges offers a place for visitors to walk mindfully and prayerfully. Two Native American medicine circles created and blessed in ceremony by a native shaman provide spaces for prayer, ceremony, and teaching. Tibetan prayer flags and prayer wheels disperse prayers to the four directions.

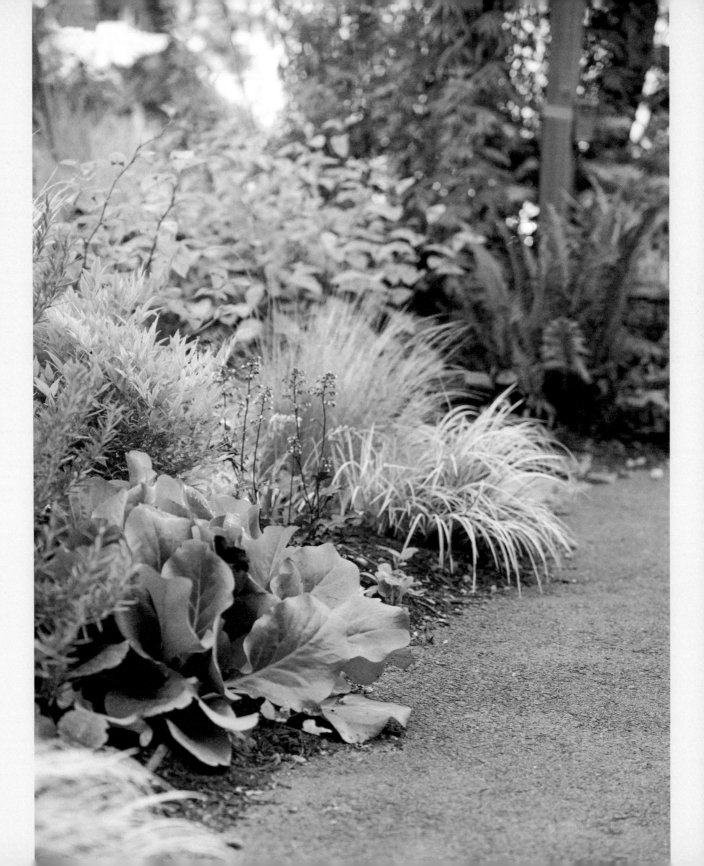

Five Steps To Creating Your Sanctuary Garden

Every garden has the potential to be a sanctuary to those who are stewarding it.

It has been said that when we heal the earth, we heal ourselves. The process of taking your sanctuary ideas off the page and beginning to shape your space to match your vision may involve some restoration work, and this work can be restorative to you, too. If the space is full of diseased or overgrown plants or has been paved over with asphalt or concrete so that the earth can barely breathe, you must first and foremost take care of restoring the earth to an ecologically robust state.

This chapter assumes that at least some aspects of your backyard ecosystem will need to be restored to health, even if you don't need to start from scratch in creating your sanctuary garden. The steps in either case are the same:

1 Clear out the space.

2 Improve the soil.

3 Manage the water.

4 Provide wildlife habitat.

5 Build the plant layers.

Step 1: Clear Out the Space

The first step in creating a sacred space is clearing it of anything that might keep you from feeling calm and at peace there. I recommend taking some time to evaluate the space with fresh eyes, as if seeing it for the first time. Take notice of anything that's not needed or that's visually distracting. This includes plants that are sick and materials that may be in the way of creating the space you envision. Bothersome objects can include old fencing, knickknacks, chipped old pots, or containers that are mismatched. Remove anything that will make you feel like you should be taking care of it, fixing it up, or otherwise dealing with it instead of meditating or relaxing.

I often find that when my clients live with a space for a long time, it becomes hard for them to imagine what it could look or feel like without all those familiar-but-ramshackle plants or objects. As you evaluate each object or plant, ask yourself when the last time was you stopped to enjoy it–or even noticed it. If you can't answer, clear it out.

PLANT ORPHANS

Deciding to remove plants can be hard for those of us who are empathetic and sensitive to ending a life. Sometimes plants require minor restoration pruning to return them to earlier glory or health, but sometimes plants are beyond repair and would rather be put out of their misery. Some plants have major wounds, some have structural issues that are dangerous or will be soon, some have been so repeatedly malpruned that they might just die of shame. As an arborist, I have seen many trees treated poorly as a common practice, whether topping them for a better view or malpruning because they are seen as a nuisance. Plants age like we do, and while some live longer than our lifetime, not all do. Plants have hormones and the ability to be restored to better health, but it can often take more resources than the steward can offer.

Over the years I have come across thousands of plants that clients wanted to get rid of for various reasons: maybe it was growing too big for the spot where it was originally planted, maybe the flowers were the wrong color, or maybe it was in a spot slated for a more desirable plant. Many people struggle with the guilt of uprooting a plant, but sometimes the space is just too valuable to let it stay. I too hate uprooting perfectly healthy plants without having a new home waiting. I have always had a plant orphanage, where all the plants I've had to move or that I simply don't want anymore come to live until they get a chance at a new beginning in a new garden.

That said, I should admit that some of my favorite plants are ones that had been slated for removal but somehow redeemed themselves. Once I told a fig that had been barren for nearly a decade that it was going to go if it didn't produce soon, and the next year it was covered in fruit!

If plants you want to remove are salvageable, consider transplanting them to a new area of your yard or giving them to friends, family, a school, or a community group that may want or need plants for a project. Good plants should not go to waste! I think you'll be surprised at how many people will step forward to take unwanted plants if you just start asking.

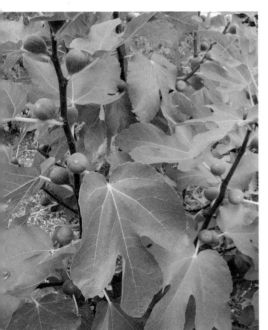

Regarded as a symbol of fertility, love, and enlightenment, the fig has been a sacred tree throughout history in many cultures.

Even common plants will be welcomed by nonprofit organizations or new gardeners who have no plants to start with or have a small budget. Donated plants can make a huge difference to them.

A number of plant species were overplanted in a certain era of landscaping and take well to transplanting. These include rhododendrons, boxwoods, roses, lilacs, nandinas, and ornamental grasses. Plants' genetic predispositions, which determine size as well as soil and water needs, can help us determine if another site is suitable for relocation. Transplanting a mature plant can be a wonderful way to add instant life to a space, and its new owners may give it that extra little boost of love it needs to be a much happier plant.

Should this plant stay or go?

Before ripping out a plant to redesign or reconfigure a garden space, consider the plant's age, what it offers, and its ecological success. Here are some questions to ask to determine if a plant should stay or go:

* Can the plant be moved elsewhere in the garden?

* Approximately how old is the plant? The younger it is, the better it may take to transplanting. The older it is, the more value it brings to the landscape, especially trees.

* Does the plant rely on support or resources (irrigation, fertilization, and such) from its people to survive?

* Does it block views or enhance them?

* Does it provide needed shade in a sunny area? Or does it shade an area where you'd like to grow sun-loving plants?

* Does it provide food for pollinators or other wildlife?

* Does it make you happy?

* What does this plant need to be happy and healthy?

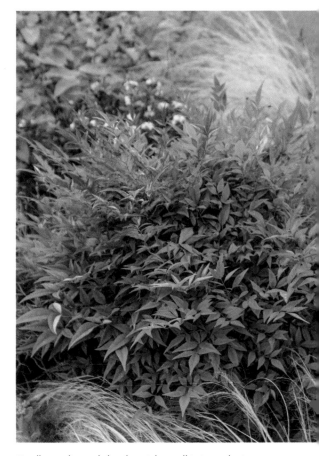

Nandina, or heavenly bamboo, takes well to transplanting and is among my favorite plants to use for good luck. Planting them near a home's entrance is said to prevent negative energy or spirits from entering the home.

FIRE AS TRANSFORMER

Fire is a sure way to create transformation in any space. In fact, it is one of nature's ways of disinfecting. In many ecosystems, it jump-starts growth and helps certain types of plants germinate. Fires are now being used in restoration projects as a way to kick-start an ecosystem and also to reduce the intensity of wildfires by burning away flammable undergrowth in advance. We can use fire to clear a space, to control unwanted vegetation, and to accomplish a general—or emotional—transformation.

A flame weeder is one handy way to use fire for weed control or prevention. When weeds have gone to seed for multiple seasons, it may be hard to get them under control so you can start over in creating your sanctuary. A flame weeder is a small torch used to burn weeds and seeds in the top layers of the soil. This method doesn't work with certain types of plants, and you'll have to be careful in dry conditions. It's always a good idea to keep a hose handy!

Smudging is a very controlled use of fire to transform the energies in a space by burning sacred herbs. It involves gathering and binding dried plant material into a smudge stick, igniting the stick and then blowing it out, and wafting the smoke from the smoldering herbs around an area. While smudging is a fairly simple ritual, you need to be careful, as the smoke can get intense if too much plant material is burning, and you could set off fire alarms if you're doing it indoors.

Smudging is traditionally used by indigenous peoples to clear negative energy from a place and cleanse one's own spirit. It is a good way to clear a space after a negative incident or interaction like an argument or when you are new to a space and want a clean slate. The scent of the smoke can be very grounding and can calm your nervous system. Besides, smudging can actually cleanse the air of harmful germs. A study published in 2007 in the *Journal of Ethnopharmacology* entitled "Medicinal Smoke Reduces Airborne Bacteria" found that burning a mixture of wood and medicinal herbs for an hour in a closed room reduced the number of airborne bacteria detected by 94 percent!

To make smudge sticks, first collect a generous handful of herbs—ones you've grown, ones that grow wild in your neighborhood, ones you purchase at the health food store or farmers' market. You'll want to use whole leaves and stems. White sage is the herb most commonly used for smudging, but there are many others, and you can make your own custom mix to fit your purposes. Here are a few herbs to consider:

* cedar–cleansing and purifying; protects from unwanted influences

* juniper–protective and cleansing; invokes abundance

* lavender–calming and relaxing; invites restful sleep

* lemon balm–cleansing and calming

* mugwort–protective, purifying, and calming; produces lucid dreams

* peppermint–protective, purifying, and refreshing; facilitates release and renewal

* pinyon pine–cleansing, healing, and strengthening

* rosemary–inspiring and invigorating; clears negativity

* sage (there are many varieties, but common culinary sage works fine)–grounding and cleansing; helps with grief

* sweetgrass–healing and purifying; invokes love, kindness, and honesty

Bundle your smudge plants in a wand and use hemp or cotton twine to wrap the plant material. Place in a dry

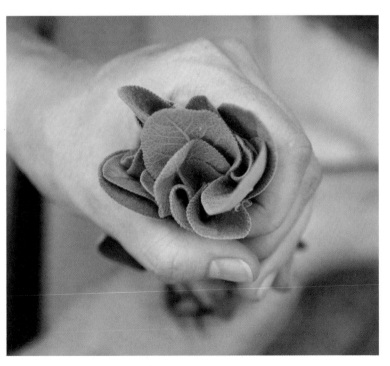

Gather the herbs in a bundle that loosely fits into your gently closed fist. An inch or two in diameter is plenty.

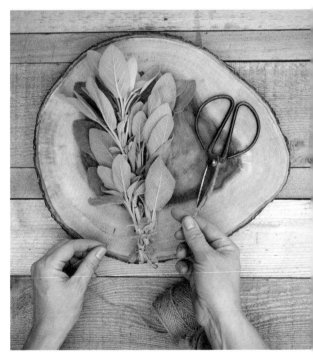

Using biodegradable twine or string, tie a knot at the bottom of your smudge stick.

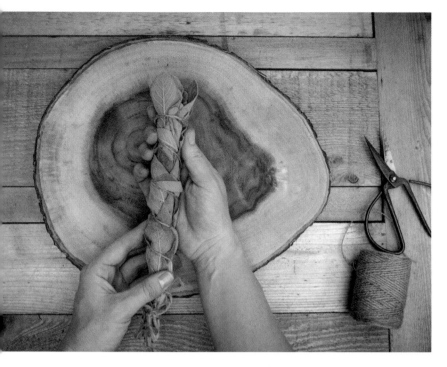

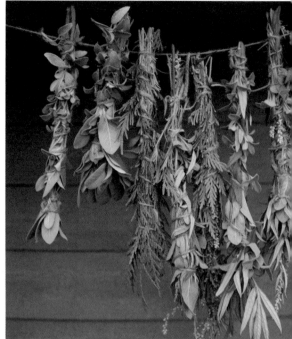

Keeping a firm grip on the plant material, wrap the twine or string around the smudge stick and tie it off at the top.

ABOVE RIGHT Hang the new smudge stick inside, preferably somewhere out of direct sunlight.

RIGHT Once the plant material is dried, light the end over a noncombustible container and blow it out to get the smudge started.

OPPOSITE Gently direct the smoke with a feather.

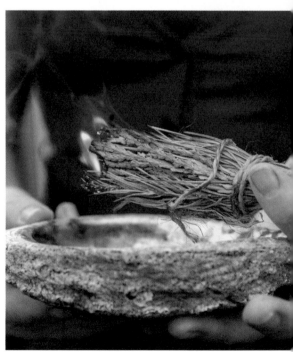

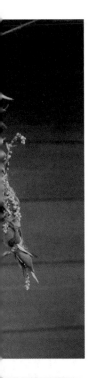

and dark area to dry the plant material completely.

Use a shell or noncombustible container to hold your smudge stick as you light it, and allow its ashes to collect in the holder. Light the smudge stick enough to see a flame, then blow out the flame so the plant material is smoldering slightly. Use a feather or your hand to fan the smoke toward yourself and then the space you want to cleanse. I start with myself outside of the space before I enter it, then circle through the space in one direction, ending where I started.

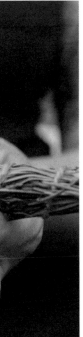

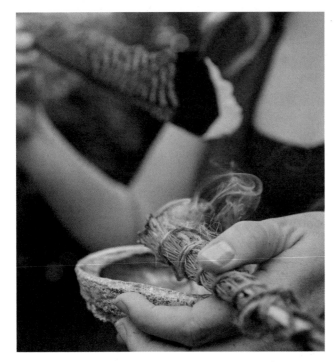

Step 2: Improve the Soil

Healthy soil is rich with life and abundant in biodiversity. One teaspoon of healthy soil contains more microbes than humans on this planet (according to soil-net.com). But most of the building sites we encounter in residential or suburban areas have been stripped of that soil long ago, to be replaced with compacted fill or soils damaged by chemical use. To take care of the earth in your sacred space, you must start with the soil and heal this ecological layer so it can function.

It can take thousands of years for healthy soil to be created naturally, but you can also build healthy, rich topsoil through these organic practices:

❋ Mulch, mulch, mulch. Use organic matter and biomass—straw, leaves, manures, and wood chips—to build the topsoil layers. Mulching with organic matter adds nutrients to the soil and can make a big difference in making your sanctuary sustainable. Mulch conserves soil moisture so you can water less often, minimizes weed growth, reduces erosion, keeps plant roots cool in summer and warm in winter, and makes your space more attractive.

❋ Cover the ground with plants. A disturbed ecosystem will grow pioneer species as a way to heal the soil naturally. Gardeners generally know these as weeds, and they can be left as a ground cover, or you can choose the plants for that job. Ground covers essentially act as a living mulch, helping to protect the soil, crowd out weeds, and build new layers of biomass every year.

☀ Tread lightly. The compaction caused by foot traffic alone can be very damaging to your soil as you try to rejuvenate and repair it.

You can use a method known as sheet mulching to quickly transform the look and health of your sacred space.

Sheet mulching is a great way to build soil and prepare new spaces.

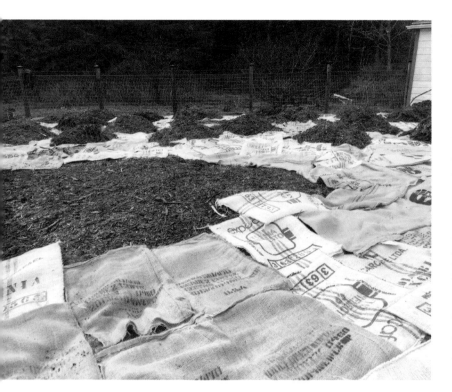

Cover the earth with a biodegradable material (cardboard and burlap are my favorites) to smother grass or weeds. On top of the material, add another layer (or two or three) of organic matter. Over time the underlying grass or weeds will decompose and enrich the soil.

Step 3: Manage the Water

Water is an essential element for all of life and thus is sacred. It nourishes the plants and can provide habitat for precious fauna. You want the sanctuary you create to use water responsibly and to use only as much as necessary. You also want to ensure that the space will not add pollutants to the water, whether it be sediments in runoff or pesticides and fertilizers that are carried into the underground aquifer.

To work with any site, to honor its natural ecological cycles and help plant life thrive sustainably, it is important to understand its hydrological state throughout the seasons. First study how much rain falls naturally. Then ask yourself how you can capture and use that water to nourish your plants and the fauna that are invited into the space or may be passing by.

Rainfall is the most natural source of water you can use in your sanctuary garden. Ideally all rainfall would be absorbed into the soil where it lands,

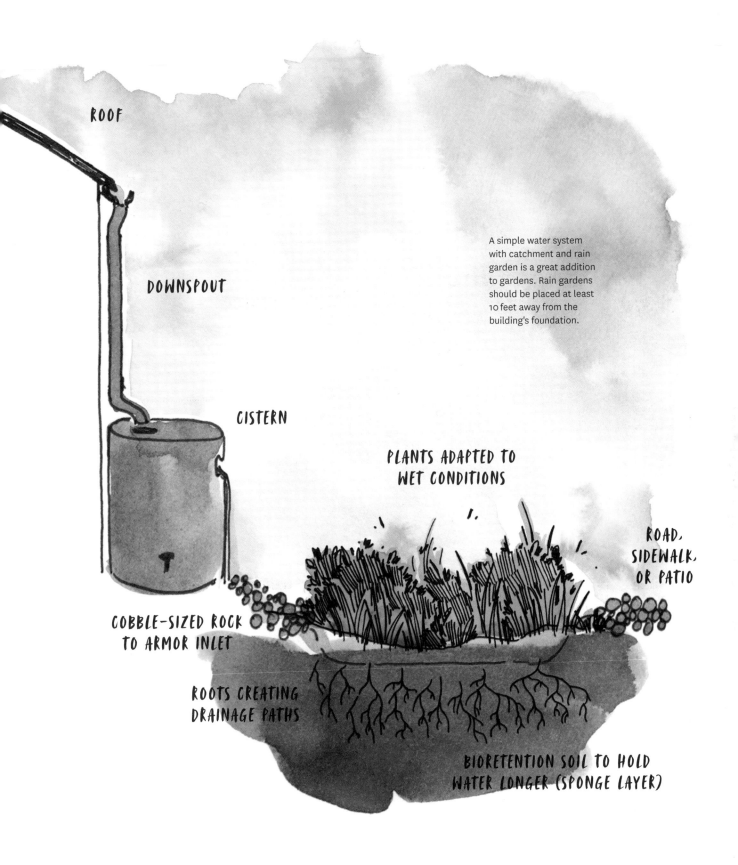

ROOF

DOWNSPOUT

CISTERN

A simple water system with catchment and rain garden is a great addition to gardens. Rain gardens should be placed at least 10 feet away from the building's foundation.

PLANTS ADAPTED TO WET CONDITIONS

ROAD, SIDEWALK, OR PATIO

COBBLE-SIZED ROCK TO ARMOR INLET

ROOTS CREATING DRAINAGE PATHS

BIORETENTION SOIL TO HOLD WATER LONGER (SPONGE LAYER)

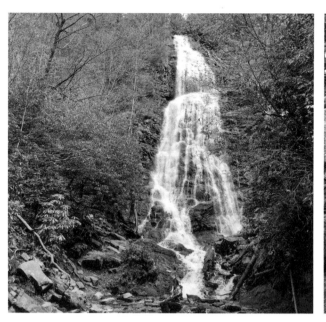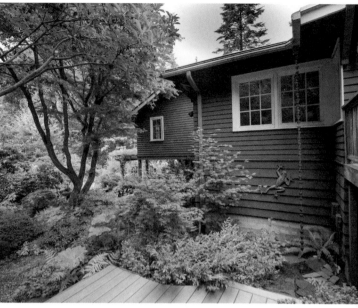

An important part of creating sanctuary is learning about the natural hydrology of your site and how it relates to the larger watershed.

ABOVE RIGHT This rain garden handles the runoff from the roof of the house and creates habitat for wildlife.

but what often happens is that impervious surfaces like rooftops, streets, and driveways shed the rain and funnel it into stormwater that causes problems downstream. As you think about managing water in your garden space, consider what happens to the stormwater if it is beyond the site's capacity to absorb it. You can use catchment methods such as barrels and cisterns to collect rainfall off of roofs or impervious surfaces. You can also create rain gardens, depressions in the landscape that collect water and slowly release it back into the soil.

A rain garden holds bioretention soil, a custom mixture of compost, sand, and loam determined by native soil and drainage rates that acts as a sponge holding the moisture. Think of the soil layer

you might find on a forest floor. Planted in the bioretention soil are species that absorb water and grow roots that create drainage channels through the new soil mix into the native soil. The inlet is the point at which water enters, either through a pipe or a trench. It is a good idea to use cobble-sized rock to armor the inlet as a way to prevent erosion. The overflow outlet is the point at which water can escape in the event that the rainwater exceeds the capacity of the pond. The outlet should be armored with rock and lead to an area with the capacity to handle excessive runoff.

For sources of more information about where to site a rain garden, how big to make it, and what to plant there, see "Further Reading and Resources."

Step 4: Provide Wildlife Habitat

Sanctuary should extend to all of the earth's inhabitants. If your goal is to live in harmony with your environment, it is essential that you consider the needs of all other beings that will pass through a space you consider sacred. Birds, bees, lizards, nematodes, and a million more life forms all have their jobs and do their part in keeping the ecosystem balanced. Birds help control pest populations and add song and beauty. Pollinators help plants to reproduce, creating fruit and food sources for other fauna. Domesticated animals all have their jobs, too, whether it is to digest biomass and cycle nutrients from one area to another or to provide us with companionship, food, fibers, or transportation.

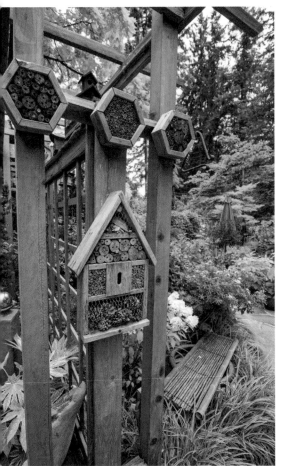

Insect hotels can house a variety of insects—especially in the winter months—by offering a range of materials that they would naturally nest in.

Providing habitat for wildlife will make your sacred space that much more fulfilling and meaningful. Be sure to include these elements:

* Native plants. Plants adapted to a specific place are going to attract the fauna adapted to that place and require less care than plants imported from elsewhere. This makes for the most resilient ecosystem.

* Biodiversity. The more plant species you have in a space, the more resilient your landscape will be and the more insect and animal species will benefit.

* Water. All living things require this essential element. In times of drought or freezing conditions, it becomes especially important for all fauna to have access to clean drinking water.

* Shelter and nesting sites. All critters need a place to raise their young. Insects need debris and biomass, pollinators need plants to feed from, and bird parents need a safe home to raise a new generation. Be sure to leave the leaves!

* Rocks. Insects and amphibians can find homes in piles of rocks.

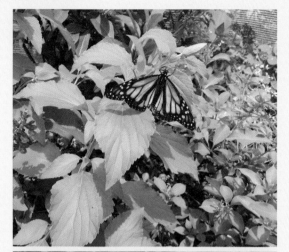

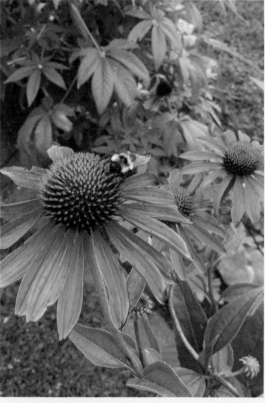

Echinacea provides color and welcomes pollinators.

TOP Pollinators appreciate a diversity of plant and flower types.

How to attract pollinators

Pollinators play many critical roles in our ecosystems, but they could use our help. Bees, butterflies, moths, beetles, flies, bats, and hummingbirds help keep insect populations in check and are responsible for a large percentage of our food supply since they help cross-pollinate plants, but their habitat is being destroyed and they are suffering from chemical use and climate change. We can invite these delicate allies into our gardens by creating habitat specifically to entice them. A few simple rules of thumb:

* Plant nectar-producing flowers for each season.

* Avoid hybridized cultivars with specialized blossoms.

* Do not use chemicals in the garden.

The best pollinator plants are natives that vary from region to region, but here are a dozen that can be grown almost anywhere:

* alstroemeria
* aster
* bee balm
* blanketflower
* borage
* butterfly weed
* cosmos
* echinacea (coneflower)
* lavender
* sweet alyssum
* penstemon
* salvia
* yarrow

You can find useful guides to pollinator plants for different regions of the country on the Xerces Society website at xerces.org/pollinator-conservation/plant-lists/ and on the Pollinator Partnership website at pollinator.org/guides.htm.

Step 5: Build the Plant Layers

A mature natural landscape typically consists of a layered community of plants, all working together in harmony to support a large, stable ecosystem. Tall canopy trees rise above shorter trees, shrubs, and herbaceous perennials. Ground covers carpet the soil. Vines, tubers/bulbs, and fungi/mushrooms complete the tapestry. A natural community like this does not require a caretaker. Imagine that—no need for weeding, watering, and fertilizing! Isn't that what you'd like for your sanctuary? If you choose plants appropriate for your sanctuary site and plant them densely to cover every inch of soil, you will create a resilient landscape that will not require a lot of maintenance.

LAYERS IN SPACE

Genetically, each plant is unique. Each plant plays a different role in succession—that is, in the natural unfolding of when and where it would grow in the environment where it is native. Some plants known as pioneer species fill a biological niche to build soil, while others offer habitat to other species or specific symbiotic relationships. Each plant will grow to a certain size within its life span and live for a certain time period before its life ends. Looking at these ecological traits can help you understand how to layer plants in your space and what you can expect as far as how to maintain them throughout their life.

Here's a closer look at the layers:

* Woody perennials—trees, shrubs, and vines—have woody structures that do not die back from year to year and can live decades or longer. For example, some tree species have a life span of twenty-five to fifty years, while others that grow more slowly and develop stronger wood can live for hundreds of years. Vines climb whatever support they are given, whether fences or trees or trellises, and can produce food for us or provide habitat for wildlife.

* Herbaceous perennials generally die back to the ground in winter and reappear bigger and stronger year after year. Some can be short lived (only a few years) and some can live for decades, spreading their tissues and seeds, and growing new plant material every year. This layer includes herbs and medicinal plants as well as perennial vegetables like asparagus and rhubarb.

* Annuals live for one season before setting their seeds to reproduce, and then they die. Most common vegetable crops are annuals.

* Bulbs have fleshy underground storage structures that persist after the foliage and flowers have made a seasonal appearance aboveground.

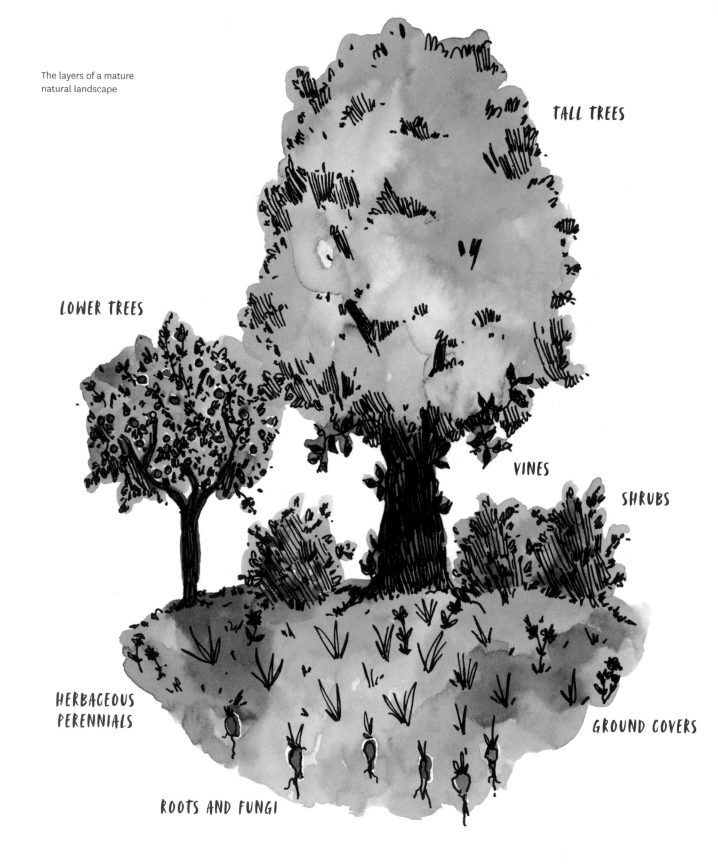

The layers of a mature natural landscape

TALL TREES

LOWER TREES

VINES

SHRUBS

HERBACEOUS PERENNIALS

GROUND COVERS

ROOTS AND FUNGI

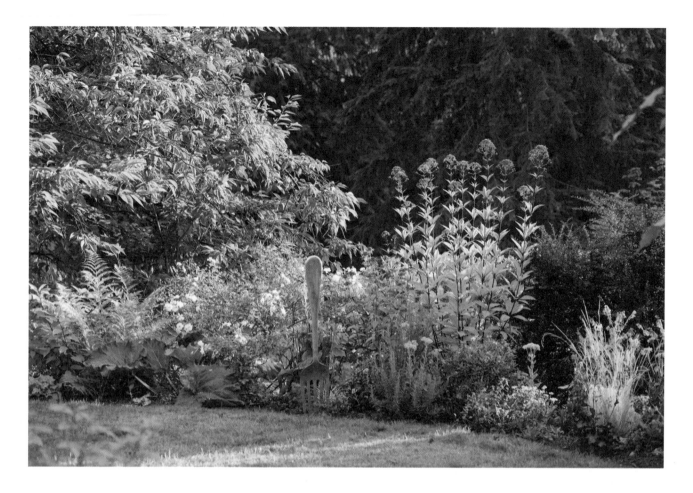

Each layer in the garden can provide multiple ecological services as well as aesthetic contrast and beauty.

❋ Fungi make up a large kingdom of organisms that are primarily known as decomposers. These often spore-bearing fruiting bodies are usually overlooked in the world of garden design and creation but can have many uses, including as food, medicine, and fibers.

Each layer of the landscape has its own natural ecological cycle, and each layer has a relationship to all the others as well. It is important to understand and honor all of these as much as possible when designing your own space. To emulate nature's harmony, start your sanctuary design with trees first and then work downward through the layers. Trees usually have the biggest visual impact, and the specimens you choose will set the stage for the rest of the landscape, depending on how they cast shade, support fauna, and release their leaves or not, and on how large they get and what their form is, whether columnar or spreading.

Based on your intentions for your sacred space, you may want to consider not

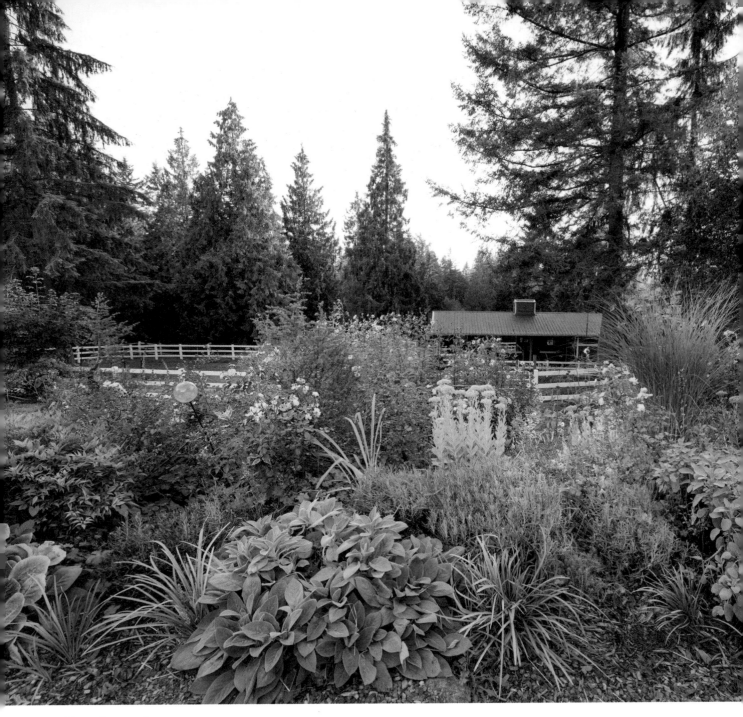

A layered community
of plants forms a stable
ecosystem that needs
little maintenance.

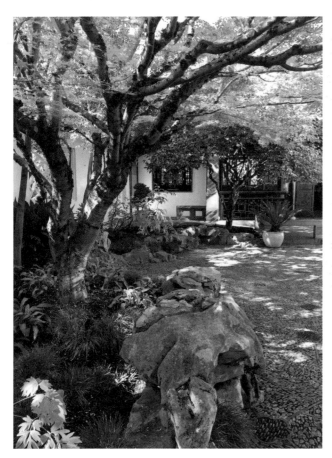

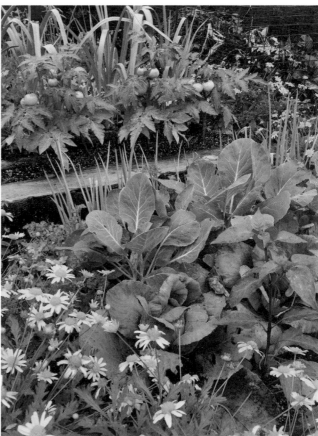

Start your sanctuary design with trees, as they have the biggest visual impact and set the stage for the rest of the landscape.

ABOVE RIGHT This layer in the garden mixes edibles with pollinator-attracting plants.

only the ecological niches plants can fill but also how plants can meet your needs for nourishment, both physical and spiritual. Incorporating edible and medicinal plants with ecologically important species as well as ornamentals gives you the best of all worlds. Sheet mulching, mentioned earlier, is a great way to prepare planting areas under trees, and you can build your layers in this way over a number of years. For instance, if you plant a new tree, you can sheet mulch around the tree and over time plant the mulched area with perennial vegetables, fruiting shrubs, and vines.

LAYERS IN TIME

Besides being layered in space, gardens are layered in time, with different species coming into leaf or bloom seasonally. Consider this aspect too as you build your sanctuary. What colors and textures would you like to see in each season? When selecting plants for your garden, it is important to plan for aesthetics as well as thinking about what uses the plants have.

Use the table to select the attributes you'd like each plant layer to provide by season so that you create a garden with

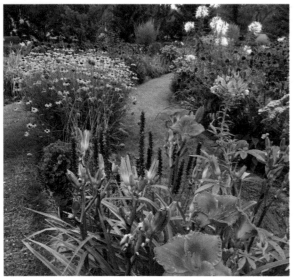

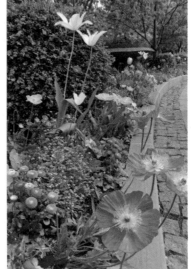

Herbaceous perennials in a Wisconsin garden include a great array of summer-flowering plants.

ABOVE RIGHT The herbaceous perennial layer in this Salt Lake City, Utah, garden provides a colorful display of spring flowers.

year-round interest. For instance, trees can offer interesting bark in the summer, blossoms in the spring, shade in the summer, and/or edibles in the fall. If you decide you want a shade tree that bears fruit and offers colorful fall foliage, you can identify species with these attributes that would work in your own area. In my area, a persimmon tree would provide those things. I generally start my designs by selecting winter attributes first and identifying plants that offer those, since it is hardest to find plants that shine in that season.

At this point you should have a good idea of the ways in which your sanctuary space can be cleared, restored, stewarded, and layered to provide for its health and your own. The next part of the book guides you in choosing specific plant allies for your sanctuary and describes some of my favorites.

What the layers can offer by season

	Trees	Shrubs	Herbaceous perennials	Tubers/ bulbs	Fungi
Winter	interesting bark	berries	seed heads for birds	edibles	ecological services
Spring	blossoms	blossoms	edibles, medicine, flowers	flowers	edibles, medicine
Summer	shade	edibles, greenery	flowers, pollinator habitat	flowers, edibles	ecological services
Fall	edibles, colorful foliage	colorful foliage	edibles, medicine	flowers, edibles	edibles, medicine

WHOLE SYSTEMS
RESEARCH FARM

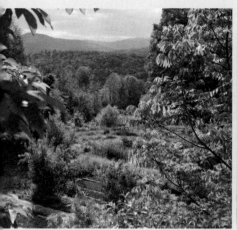
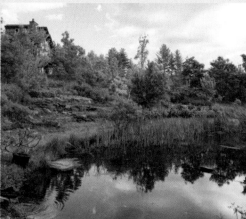
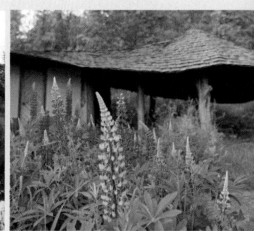

ABOVE, FROM LEFT TO RIGHT

Embodying sanctuary, Whole Systems Research Farm offers this tranquil view to the west.

On a terrace close to the home and shop is a pond central to meeting human needs as well as providing habitat for numerous species—wild and domestic.

This whimsical structure contains a wood-fired sauna and has a small pond nearby for cold plunges.

ON A WEST-FACING SLOPE in rural Vermont lies a sanctuary for times of rapid change, being developed according to permaculture principles of caring for the land. Its steward, Ben Falk, is a designer, builder, ecologist, tree-tender, and backcountry traveler. Author of *The Resilient Farm and Homestead*, he is concerned with biological and cultural extinction and the increasing separation between people and elemental things. He and his wife, Erica, a naturopathic doctor and herbalist, live on a hillside farm on 10 acres of wet field and forest in the Mad River Valley.

The farm serves as headquarters for Whole Systems Design, LLC, and hosts interns, permaculture courses, and visiting client teams. Ben and his colleagues at Whole Systems Design have been performing what they call regenerative land use experiments on the farm. In constant interaction with the land, which they consider their teacher, they have developed an edible landscape of ponds, fruit and nut trees, forest and pasture, stone and timber structures, and outdoor living spaces. Buildings include a home, a woodshop, and a whimsical sauna. The permaculture design firm consults on projects around the United States and abroad. Its mission statement is "We identify, design, and develop human habitats that yield perennial abundance and enduring value."

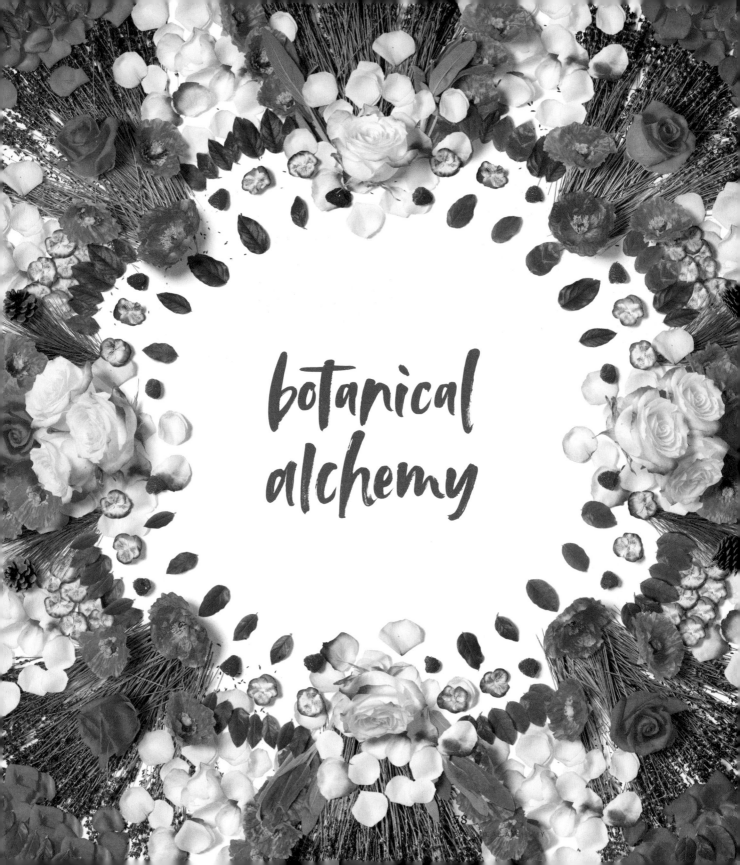

botanical
alchemy

"A plant may not talk, but there is a spirit in it that is conscious, that sees everything, which is the soul of the plant, its essence, what makes it alive."

PABLO AMARINGO, *AYAHUASCA VISIONS*

Plants are fascinating biological organisms—silent beings without which we wouldn't exist. From the beginning of human history, plants have played critical roles in our existence and evolution. We owe our lives to plants. Through gaseous exchange, they clean the air and essentially breathe without lungs. They convert sunlight into sugars, feeding themselves and those around them. They transfer nutrients, minerals, and fluids through their tissues, without organs to aid in pumping such materials, sometimes hundreds of feet upward into the sky. They then turn those valuable resources into foods, medicine, and materials we can use. The alchemy of plants is mesmerizing.

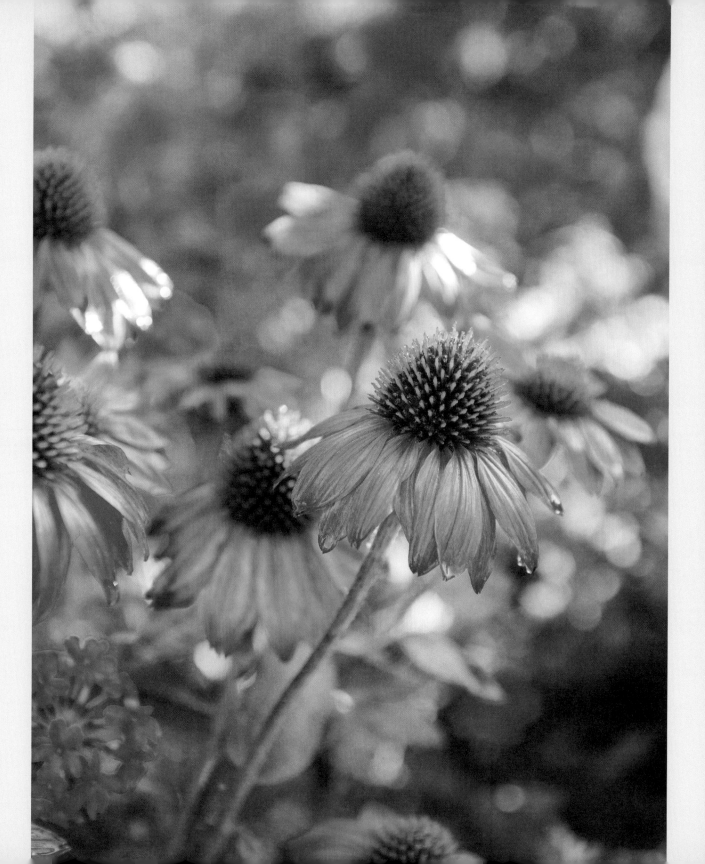

I've felt a deep love for plants as far back as I can remember. I recall speaking to them as a young child, offering to help spread the seeds of tall meadow grasses and sitting with wise old trees to feel comforted. They were all friends to me and continue to be. As a young adult, I studied plants with tenacity: memorizing botanical names, calculating growth, smelling and tasting foliage and flowers, imagining how their colors and textures would play well and dance with other plants—in the wind, in the snow, in the late afternoon in August. I kept samples of pressed plant parts. Before long, my entire world was immersed in the plant kingdom. That's all I would see and think about. When I'd learn about a new plant, I'd ask, How can that plant be used in my garden? I studied the science of plants for years, getting every credential needed, becoming certified as a horticulturalist and arborist. But ultimately what I found is that you cannot learn everything there is to know about plants from a book or in school. You must spend time in their presence to get to know their spirits and the gifts they offer.

Echinacea offers us healing gifts, and it also nourishes other life forms such as birds, bees, and soil organisms.

As you think about the plants that will be part of your sanctuary, consider how they can help you on your quest for health and well-being. Plant medicine can cure physical ills as well as emotional and spiritual ailments. Plants can help us work with focus, and they can help us relax. Plants can truly alter our spirits. If we choose to pay attention and look for new ways to interact with them, we can build relationships with plants we encounter every day. Plants become wonderful teachers offering wisdom and nourishment in many ways.

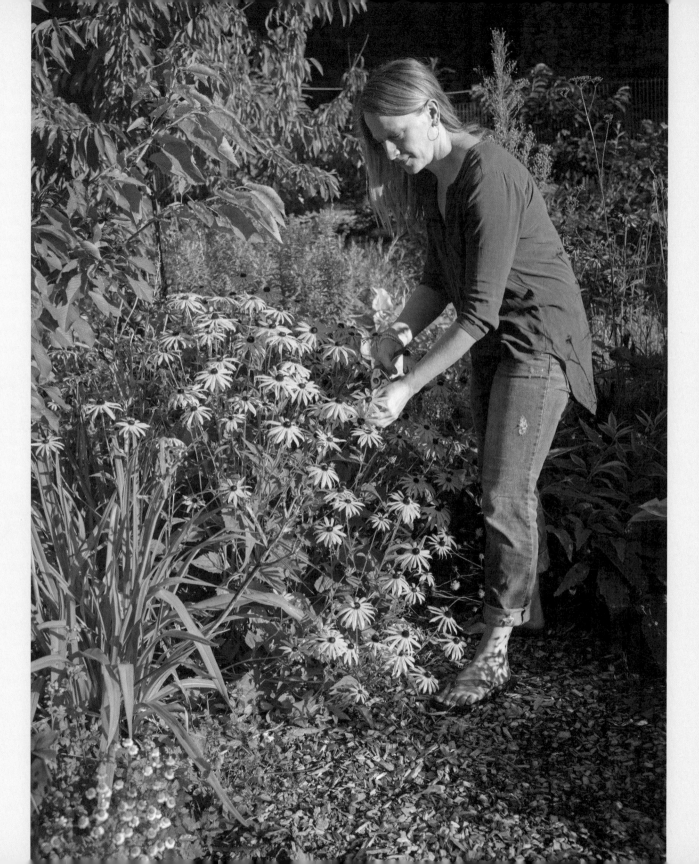

Fifty Sacred Plants for the Sanctuary Garden

If you build a relationship with each plant in your garden, you will be pleasantly surprised to learn of its many uses.

In the following pages, I profile my top fifty plant picks for sanctuary spaces, both for building the layers and for building potentially healing relationships with. These are plants that have important ecological functions and are easy to find and grow. They also have a long history of human use for medicinal and other purposes, and they have sacred powers that have been told in myths and stories that have accompanied them down through the ages. They are well worth getting to know from these multiple perspectives.

The plant profiles are organized by forest layer—trees, vines, shrubs, herbaceous perennials, and annuals. This list is by no means exhaustive and is meant to stimulate your own curiosity and motivate you to research plants that interest you. If one plant calls to you, there is usually a reason. Subsequent chapters will guide you in developing a relationship with the plants you choose for your sanctuary and making use of them beyond the functions they serve in the garden ecosystem.

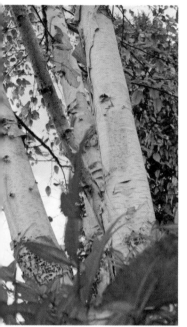

BIRCH

Betula species

GROWTH HABIT upright, deciduous trees or shrubs, 40–70 feet tall SACRED POWERS renews, cleanses, builds courage, offers protection

Best known for their striking white bark, birches include many deciduous hardwood trees and shrubs. Ecologically, they are a pioneer species that grows quickly and are often found in lowlands or near wetlands; they are easily stressed by drought. The wood has been used for centuries as firewood and construction material, and the skinlike bark can be used for paper. The bark and small green leaves contain plentiful oils, and the tree produces a medicinal sap that is rich in fructose. Beverages and syrup made from the sap can help with a wide variety of ailments, including kidney stones, digestive issues, and respiratory problems. To make a simple medicinal tea, use a few fresh leaves in spring and pour boiling water over them, steeping for five to ten minutes. In ancient Siberia and Europe, this tree was considered sacred. Birches symbolize new beginnings, and the birch is the tree for the first month in the Celtic calendar.

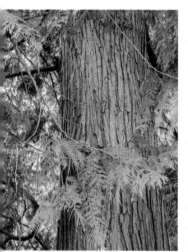

Western red cedar
(*Thuja plicata*)

CEDAR

Various species and common names

GROWTH HABIT evergreen conifers, 70–100 feet tall SACRED POWERS helps cleanse or purify and confer protection

Many trees known as cedars grow throughout the world; they vary in genus and species and grow to a range of sizes. Some examples are deodar cedar (*Cedrus deodara*), western red cedar (*Thuja plicata*), arborvitea (*Thuja occidentalis*), Port Orford cedar (*Chamaecyparis lawsoniana*), and yellow cedar (*Callitropsis nootkatensis*). All cedars are evergreen conifers with fanlike or scalelike needles. All cedars contain powerful antimicrobial and antifungal agents, making cedar a prized rot-resistant material for building. With their aromatic properties, they are used in aromatherapy and incense; the oils also have an insecticidal effect and are safe insect repellents. Other medicinal uses include as an expectorant, a cleanser, and a diuretic. Cedar oil can be used in a respiratory steam and in tinctures, salves, and infused oils. Considered sacred by Native Americans and one of the four sacred plants used in ceremony, the cedar is known as the tree of life.

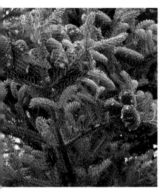

FIR

Abies species

GROWTH HABIT symmetrical evergreen conifers, 40–60 feet tall SACRED POWERS represents clear vision, higher perspectives, youthfulness

Firs include several dozen species of evergreen conifers in the pine family, all growing in the Northern Hemisphere in middle to upper elevations. Their needles are usually flat, and cones differ from other conifers in that they are held vertical to the branches, much like candles. The sap from the tree is sticky and has been used as a glue or to help hold bandages in place; it can also be made into a healing ointment or salve for the skin. Essential oil from the balsam fir is a popular fragrance and is used in aromatherapy to help fight fatigue, keep a person grounded, uplift the mind, and relax the body. The needles can be used in a tea to help treat a number of illnesses—respiratory ailments, sore throats, and even headaches.

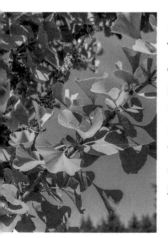

GINKGO

Ginkgo biloba

OTHER COMMON NAMES maidenhair tree, ancestor tree, eyes of the cosmic spirit tree, Buddha's fingernail tree GROWTH HABIT deciduous pyramidal to upright oval, 70–100 feet tall SACRED POWERS represents survival and adaptability; associated with prosperity, longevity, health, and fertility

The ginkgo tree has existed since prehistoric times, with fossils dating back 300 million years. These trees can grow large and live for a thousand years or more. Many elders of the species live in Buddhist temples in Asia, where they are protected as sacred. Once nearly extinct, they have made a resurgence in horticulture, and in urban settings as they have

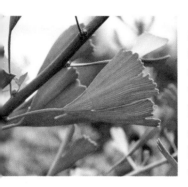

proven their resilience in the face of environmental toxins, even surviving radiation from the Hiroshima atomic bombing. The ginkgo tree enjoys soils with moisture but also adequate drainage, making it a great tree for riparian areas. Ginkgo leaves have a very distinct two-lobed pattern and turn a radiant gold in autumn, a color retained even after the tree has dropped the leaves in a glowing circle around it. Females of the species produce seeds with skins that emit an unpleasant odor. Chinese medicine makes extensive use of ginkgo seeds in herbal formulas to treat asthma, bronchitis, and vaginal discharge. In western medicine, the leaf is well known for protecting and enhancing brain function and is often prescribed to aid the vascular or circulatory system, for age-related memory ailments, and to help with premenstrual syndrome, attention deficit hyperactivity disorder, and depression. My own experience with ginkgo is that it cleans up any cobwebs in my brain.

HAWTHORN

Crataegus species

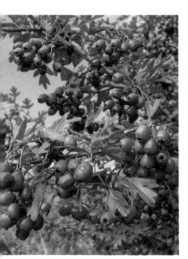

OTHER COMMON NAMES thornapple, May-tree, hawberry, whitethorn GROWTH HABIT deciduous pyramidal trees and shrubs to 35 feet tall SACRED POWERS protects and cleanses the grieving heart

This genus includes both trees and shrubs. All grow thorns and produce spring flowers followed by a small rosaceous fruit. The plant grows well in many conditions and works well in hedgerows. Ecologically, it provides habitat for a large variety of species and serves as an important food source in winter. Known as a medicinal plant in ancient Greece, it was prescribed as a heart medicine and is still used today for numerous heart-related ailments, with studies to back up its effectiveness. Its young leaves and berries, also called haws, are edible, and dried haws have been used in Chinese medicine as a digestive aid. Hawthorn is one of the trees in the Celtic calendar and is said in Celtic and Gaelic folklore to be a sacred tree for fairies and witches. Being at the peak of its bloom around May 1, hawthorn has long been associated with Beltane (May Day) and the beginnings of spring. The Celts would festoon the entrances to their homes and stables with blossoming branches of hawthorn to welcome in the warmer months.

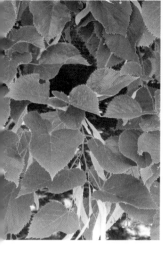

LINDEN

OTHER COMMON NAMES lime tree, basswood GROWTH HABIT deciduous pyramidal to upright oval, 60–70 feet tall SACRED POWERS calms the heart, brings good fortune, and helps with feeling vibrant

Lindens are large trees with heart-shaped leaves that are commonly found in urban areas as street trees thanks to their adaptability. The trees provide dense shade and can grow in a wide range of conditions.

Ecologically, their flowers are an important nectar source for bees. I've affectionately called my linden tree the Salad Tree, making a ritual out of harvesting its young leaves in spring as a replacement for annual greens in meals. Medicinally, the flower is used in herbal remedies and teas for relaxing the nervous system and high blood pressure, among other healing purposes. The leaves can be used as a poultice to treat wounds.

OAK

Quercus species

GROWTH HABIT deciduous or evergreen shrubs and trees up to 140 feet tall SACRED POWERS symbolizes strength, courage, ancient knowledge; considered an entryway or threshold to the great mysteries of life

Oak trees and shrubs span the globe in the Northern Hemisphere, producing distinctly lobed leaves and acorns. The strong wood of the oak has been used for framing and building from before the Vikings used it in their ships in the ninth century. Oaks are elders, and ecologically they are keystone species living in a number of different conditions, but oak species have declined due to pests, disease, and climate change. The tree hosts more than two thousand insect species and

many mammal and bird species. Acorns are rich in nutrients, minerals, fats, and carbohydrates and are a great food source for many animals. The tannins, however, can be toxic to ruminants such as cattle, sheep, goats, and horses when eaten in excess. Medicinally, oak bark has been used as an astringent and can be made into a tea or used in bathing, compresses, ointments, and tinctures applied externally. Spiritually, oaks are most sacred to the Celts and Druids, but they are also greatly respected in the myths of many ancient cultures; the oak was the tree of the god Zeus. The tree has played an important role in ceremony and ritual space, and in the fairy realm is considered to host many spirits.

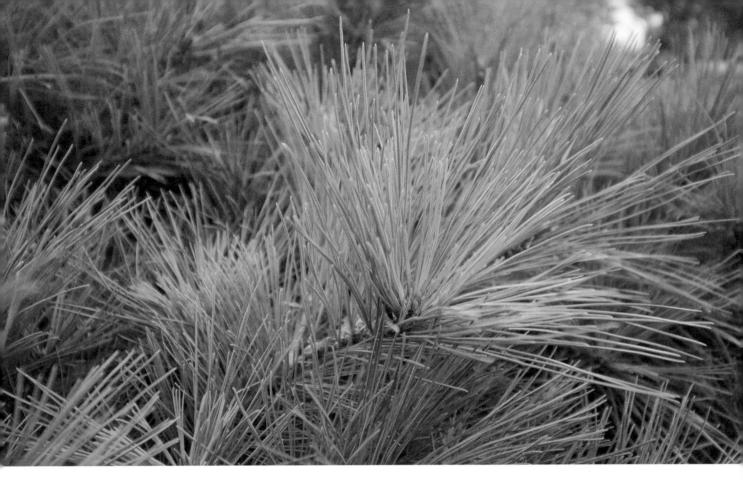

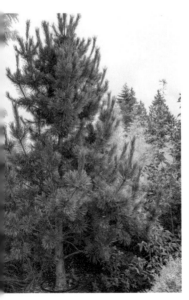

PINE

Pinus species

GROWTH HABIT evergreen conifers up to 100 feet tall SACRED POWERS helps restore a positive emotional state, takes away guilt, and symbolizes renewal, humbleness, vitality, and prosperity

More than a hundred species of pine are found throughout the world, with ancestors from the Jurassic era. They typically do best in acidic soils and difficult growing conditions. An important lumber crop today, this tree has also been a food source and was historically an important source of vitamin C. Well known as a cleansing agent, the oil can be added to homemade deodorant, cleaning, or air-freshening products or used as incense. Pine needle tea can uplift your spirits and clear your mind. Pine is one of the seven chieftain trees of the Irish (totems for clans) and is mentioned in Roman mythology.

WILLOW

Salix species

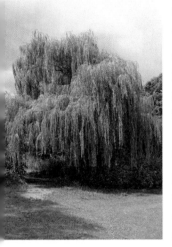

GROWTH HABIT deciduous, spreading, weeping shrubs and trees up to 65 feet tall
SACRED POWERS represents flexibility, emotional healing, protection, regrowth

One of my favorite trees, this beauty has grace and an enchanting history from cultures all around the world. The genus *Salix* includes more than four hundred species, from large trees to small shrubs and even small sprawling ground covers. They enjoy growing in moist soils and have a fast growth rate, absorbing minerals and nutrients quickly, making them great for ecological restoration of degraded wetlands and riparian areas. Their roots can be invasive in residential settings, though, clogging pipes. Willow is best known medically as the source of salicylic acid, which is what the anti-inflammatory drug aspirin is made from, and its medical uses have been documented since the fifth century BC. It is a sacred tree in many religions—including Judaism, Christianity, Buddhism, Taoism, and Paganism—and is used in ceremonies and as a subject of folklore around the world. It is also one of the thirteen trees in the Celtic calendar.

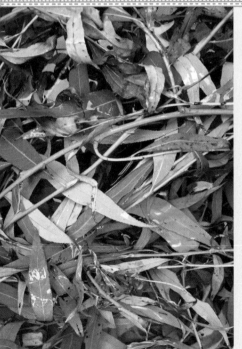

Make a potion to grow new plants

The branches of willow contain a rooting hormone that aids root development and growth in plants. The medicinal properties of willow help the new seedling or rooted plant stay healthy and often grow at a quicker rate. Simply take cuttings of a willow—fresh tips are the best—and place 1-inch lengths in a jar, cover with cool water, and let them sit in the sun for a few days. Then drain the water into another jar and place in that jar cuttings of plants you want to propagate, leaving them to soak overnight before planting. You can also use this potion to water a planting medium you've placed your cuttings in. Two waterings should be enough to give the cuttings a little boost.

Making willow potion is simple, with only two ingredients: willow and water.

VINES

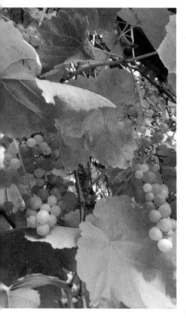

GRAPE

Vitis species

GROWTH HABIT clings with tendrils on stems up to 115 feet long SACRED POWERS symbolizes fertility and prosperity; brings good fortune

This woody vine has been cultivated for its fruit throughout the world for more than seven thousand years. The plant enjoys sunshine, well-drained soil, and support from an arbor or sturdy structure, as it gets heavy and grows fast. Grapes are used to produce wine, raisins, and juices, and have been touted as medicinal for thousands of years and used to treat a variety of ailments in folk medicine. Studies have proven that the resveratrol in grapes is a powerful antioxidant, protecting the body from free radicals, helping to prevent disease, and helping to maintain a healthy heart. The seed extract is now commonly used for lowering blood pressure, treating vision problems, reducing edema and weight gain, and increasing blood flow. Grapes have played a significant role in religious ritual and are mentioned in the Bible.

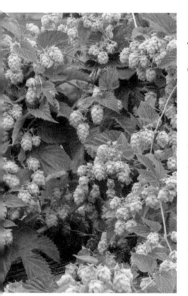

HOPS

Humulus lupulus

GROWTH HABIT climbs with stiff hairs on stems 18–25 feet long SACRED POWERS induces relaxation and aids peaceful sleep

The flower of this fast-growing perennial vine is best known as an ingredient in beer but is also a safe herb for most to ingest. Used in the brewing process since the eleventh century, hops has been a controversial and even prohibited crop at times. It likes rich soil, full sun, and some sort of structure to climb on; it grows all over several of my fences, making it easy to harvest the flowers. Medicinally, it is antibacterial and antimicrobial, and it aids digestion and sleep. Hops are easy to use in teas or tinctures, producing a mild sedative effect, and are also a bitter tonic. I like to use hops in dream pillows for their help in creating peaceful rest and find it interesting that King James III and Abraham Lincoln did the same.

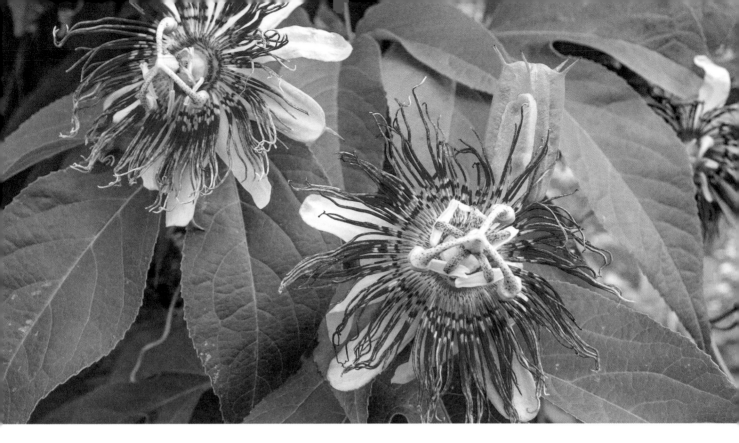

PASSIONFLOWER

Passiflora incarnata

OTHER COMMON NAMES maypop, apricot vine, passion vine **GROWTH HABIT** clings with tendrils on stems up to 10 feet long **SACRED POWERS** helps with attracting friendship and love; promotes peace

This tropical vine produces dramatic flowers with intricate details and layering. The plant is named for the passion of Christ—his sufferings in the last days before his crucifixion. Grown in warmer regions, passionflower has evolved with many other species that use it. Bats, hummingbirds, and a variety of bees and wasps pollinate it. The leaves are food and habitat for butterflies and other lepidoptera. The fruit is edible, and the entire plant is used for teas and tinctures. Indigenous Americans (north and south) have used the plant medicinally in a variety of ways, including to heal skin ailments and as a blood tonic. Passionflower is currently known as a sedative used to quell anxiety and quiet the mind. In dream pillows, it helps promote sleep and quiet dreams; in incense, it is used to promote understanding and in equinox rituals.

ELDERBERRY

Sambucus nigra

OTHER COMMON NAMES black elder, pip tree, devil's wood GROWTH HABIT deciduous shrub, 10–15 feet tall SACRED POWERS functions as a guardian if planted near the kitchen; wards off evil spirits when branches are hung

A powerful medicine, elderberry can grow in a variety of conditions in temperate regions—in sun or shade, in wet or dry soils, but it can also become weedy. It is beneficial to wildlife, providing nesting sites and food for birds and other small mammals. Livestock do not eat the stems of this plant, making it a good pasture plant for under and around large shade trees and in hedgerows. The berries have antiviral, anti-inflammatory, and antioxidant properties, which make them an effective tonic for flu and cold season. They are used in syrups, infused honeys, wines, and teas. (Caution: the red fruiting species is poisonous.) Elder flowers are used in many beverages and are known as an antihistamine effective against allergies. Mythological stories include the superstition that a spirit resides in the plant that will bring about bad luck if you damage the plant without offering any gratitude, and that if you fall asleep under an elder, you will dream of the fairy world. It was also believed that the cross of Jesus was made from elder wood.

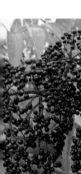
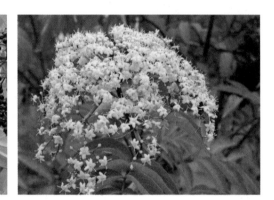

LAVENDER

Lavandula species

GROWTH HABIT evergreen shrub, 1–3 feet tall and wide SACRED POWERS helps with meditation, mental clarity, psychic development; strengthens love

This small Mediterranean herb is short lived but powerful and useful in many ways—as a medicinal, cosmetic, and culinary herb, and also as a host for beneficial insects. It prefers a sunny location and well-drained soil, making it a great addition to your drought-tolerant garden. Lavender oil can help us relax and get to sleep, and it has antidepressant properties. It can also help soothe headaches, body aches and pains, and skin problems like insect bites, burns, and rashes. It acts as a disinfectant and can be added to bath water for a relaxing effect. It is my favorite infused oil to make and have on hand. I carry lavender oil with me when I travel and use the flowers in sachets and dream pillows. Lavender is one of the holy herbs named

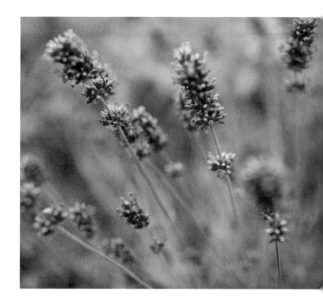

in the Bible, and it was a common plant used for cleaning in medieval times.

RASPBERRY

Rubus species

GROWTH HABIT deciduous perennial shrub, 4–5 feet tall, spreading underground
SACRED POWERS protects from unfriendly spirits and helps with matters of the heart

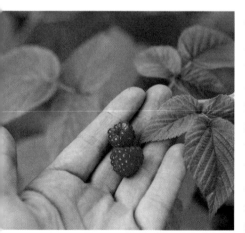

The raspberry plant is one of my favorite garden "weeds" to pull and share. Producing delicious and nutritious fruit, this plant also provides nectar, food, and shelter for wildlife. The canes can be trellised for easier harvest and production, but this is not necessary. The berries, rich in nutrients and minerals, have been considered medicinal since the Middle Ages. Raspberry leaf is best known as an astringent herb with beneficial effects on the digestive system, the throat, and women's reproductive system, making it a great addition to teas for menstrual pain relief. Many Native American tribes used the plant, including its roots, for a variety of ailments. In folklore, raspberries symbolized fertility, and raspberry leaf is a safe herb for pregnant and nursing women, with studies showing that it can ease childbirth.

ROSE

Rosa species

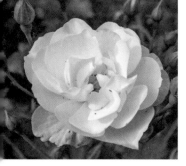

GROWTH HABIT shrubs, climbers, ground covers
SACRED POWERS as rose water, used to clean and
protect spaces and people; flowers used as
symbolic charms and of course in love spells

Oh, the beloved rose, a flower that universally represents love! This gorgeous blossom graces gardens around the world, and the genus includes hundreds of species and cultivars. Roses are prized as cut flowers and for their expensive fragrant oils used in perfume and beauty products. Most roses are edible and medicinal as well. The whole plant has been used in traditional medicine for a variety of ailments, but the petals and rose hips are most used now. The rose hips contain vitamin C and antioxidants, both used for respiratory illnesses, women's complaints, and digestive ailments. The astringent properties of roses make them good for treating insect bites, wounds, burns, and rashes, and rose water can be used as a cleanser or toner for everyday self-care. Relaxing in a bath full of rose petals and inhaling their scent can help alleviate anxiety, depression, and nervousness. Roses are also known as an aphrodisiac. Roses are common in folklore around the globe, representing and symbolizing among other things the blood of Christ, innocence, and adultery.

ROSEMARY

Rosmarinus officinalis

OTHER COMMON NAMES compass weed, sea
dew, elf leaf GROWTH HABIT evergreen shrub
up to 5 feet tall and wide SACRED POWERS used
for protection and purification; symbolizes
love, mental strength, remembrance

Rosemary is a well-known culinary herb native to the Mediterranean. Several varieties are cultivated, with different growth habits and even flower colors. With its evergreen needles, the shrub is well adapted to drought and growing in warm, dry weather. Bees love the small flowers. Rosemary has many time-honored uses as a medicine—for indigestion, for joint and muscle pain, to stimulate hair growth, and to improve circulation and memory. Studies show it can lower cortisol levels, inhibit foodborne illnesses, and quell cancerous tumor growth. This powerful herb also has an impressive history, with stories of it being used by many famous characters throughout time. Sacred to the Greeks and Egyptians, it was seen as a symbol of remembrance and fidelity and was often used in weddings, funerals, and other ceremonies. Rosemary was worn for protection during the time of the plague, and rosemary incense was believed to help purify the air in sickrooms. Its magical properties include protecting against nightmares and evil spirits. My favorite old saying about this plant is "Where rosemary flourishes, the woman rules."

SAGE

Salvia species

GROWTH HABIT evergreen or woody perennial shrub, 1–3 feet tall and wide **SACRED POWERS** used as a smudge or in incense to purify and cleanse spaces and the human spirit; used for grounding, spells of immortality, gaining wisdom, and alleviating grief (white sage)

The genus *Salvia* includes more than a thousand species. Common sage (*Salvia officinalis*) is a warming, pungent herb used mostly for culinary purposes. It prefers sunshine and well-drained soils, being a drought-tolerant plant, and is great for pollinators when it blooms in the summer. The medicinal uses date back to the Middle Ages, when sage tea was considered a health tonic. Today sage is used for upper respiratory issues (sore throats, runny noses, colds, fever), weak digestion (bloating, nausea, flatulence), and to lift depression and dark spirits. It is also known to help with pain in the joints or arthritis, especially when cold brings it on. It improves circulation, boosts insulin, helps insomnia, treats yeast infections, and can even be used as a hair rinse. A simple way to use sage is to make a tea with its leaves and add honey if the astringent taste isn't to your liking. White sage (*Salvia apiana*) grows mainly in the Southwest and is one of the sacred herbs in Native American culture, used in ceremony and as medicine.

Common sage (*Salvia officinalis*)

FAR RIGHT White sage (*Salvia apiana*)

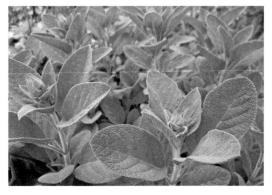

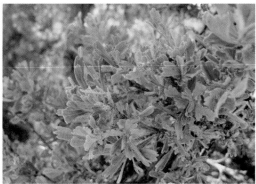

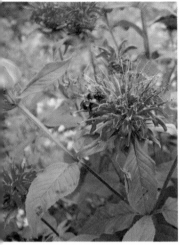

BEE BALM

Monarda didyma, M. fistulosa

OTHER COMMON NAMES Oswego tea, scarlet bergamot, mountain mint, sweet leaf GROWTH HABIT upright, to 4 feet tall, spreading through rhizomes SACRED POWERS helps us understand our passions and can help us attract the resources we need for our calling, but only if we are respectful to the earth

Bee balm is native to North America and grows well in sunny conditions, preferring a rich and moist soil. Its brightly colored flowers are a favorite of pollinators—bees, butterflies, and hummingbirds especially. The leaves and flowers contain oils with compounds having antiseptic, fungicidal, and antibiotic properties. Thymol, one of those compounds, was first discovered in 1719 and was extracted from bee balm (and thyme) but is now created synthetically in a lab. Thymol is used in a variety of ways—as a preservative, a fungicide, and a dewormer, and in mouthwashes. Several Native American tribes use the plant's medicine for ailments including colds, digestive complaints, burns, and insomnia. Modern herbalists use bee balm for the same issues. As an aromatic, it is a perfume additive and is best used fresh but can also be dried.

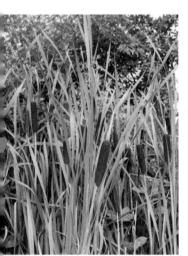

CATTAIL

Typha species

OTHER COMMON NAMES bulrush, reedmace GROWTH HABIT upright stalks, 3–10 feet tall SACRED POWERS symbolizes peace, and the flowers, prosperity

Several dozen cattail species grow around the world and are among the most useful plants that grow in wetlands or in moist soils. Cattail provides habitat for many animals and insects, colonizes quickly, and can take over an area through its spreading rhizomes or seed. It has been an important plant in many cultures, including ancient Rome and indigenous America, for its use in medicine, food, and drink, and as tinder, sealant, roofing thatch, and fiber. The protein-rich pollen is flammable, making a spark when ignited, so the plant was once used in fireworks. It is now being researched as a bioremediation plant to help clean pollutants out of water and as a feedstock for high-yielding ethanol fuel. In Chinese medicine, the pollen of cattail (Pu Huang), in capsule or poultice form, is used to stop internal and external bleeding. In Ayurvedic medicine, the rhizome is used for its diuretic and astringent properties.

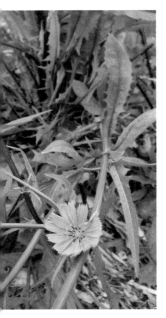

CHICORY

Cichorium species

OTHER COMMON NAMES wild succory, blue sailor, coffeeweed, wild endive, blue daisy GROWTH HABIT upright, with stems 10–40 inches tall SACRED POWERS reminds us to love unconditionally and in freedom

This herbaceous perennial with its beautiful blue flowers can be seen growing wild along roadsides in much of the world. Its deep taproot allows it to grow where other plants struggle. It is also cultivated in gardens for a number of uses—the spring leaves are edible although bitter, and the root is used medicinally. It has been used for at least two thousand years in a number of ways. Known as an antioxidant and source of vitamin C, chicory root makes a great coffee substitute without the stimulant caffeine. The root also contains inulin, which can be used as a sugar additive and soluble fiber. Chicory is being used in forage mixtures for livestock because it is resilient, provides protein, is highly palatable, and has been found in research studies to reduce internal parasites in farm animals.

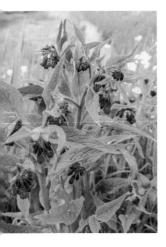

COMFREY

Symphytum species

OTHER COMMON NAMES boneknit, boneset, bruisewort, knitbone GROWTH HABIT upright, 3–4 feet tall SACRED POWERS protects travelers and aids letting go of unhealthy relationships

Comfrey is an all-star plant, capable of enriching soil and healing our bodies. This herbaceous perennial grows a deep taproot that draws up minerals and nutrients, making them available for us and other plants to use. It can grow just about anywhere and produces a large volume of hairy leaves that can be used in the compost pile, as green mulch, or as medicine, although they may require gloves to handle. Pollinators visit its bell-like flower. Known as a medicinal plant for thousands of years, comfrey contains allantoin, which is a cell proliferant, regenerating and aiding the repair of damaged tissues. It can help with almost any skin or tissue-related issue externally, as a fresh poultice, infused into oils, or made into a salve. Its edibility has been debated, as it is said to cause liver damage with ongoing consumption, but it has been used in infusions for centuries and many herbalists swear by it.

ECHINACEA

Echinacea purpurea, E. angustifolia, E. pallida

OTHER COMMON NAMES purple coneflower GROWTH HABIT upright to 4 feet tall SACRED POWERS confers inner strength, protection, and prosperity; increases potency of spells and magic

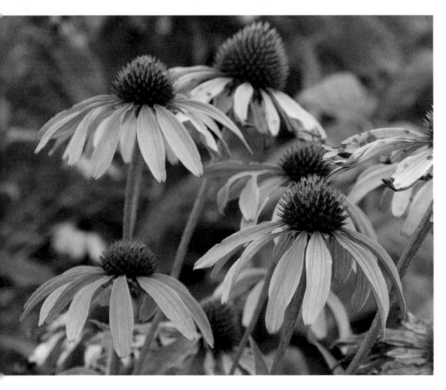

This North American native is well known as a medicine as well as being a beautiful ornamental and providing food for pollinators. Birds, bees, butterflies, and other critters all use this plant for food at different times of the year. Medicinally, native tribes across the plains used it to treat a variety of ailments, including tooth pain, fatigue, and skin conditions. Echinacea has been popularized as an herb to boost the immune system and treat the common cold by increasing white blood cells. Even though it was the most frequently used plant preparation in the United States in the early 1900s, controversy and debate exists within the scientific community about this plant's abilities as a medicine. Try chewing on a leaf or root to feel its constituents work. In the magical realm, it is believed to attract abundance, magic, and miracles. It is also regarded as an aphrodisiac, which can help increase fertility.

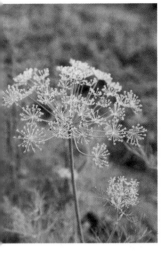

FENNEL

Foeniculum vulgare

GROWTH HABIT perennial often grown as annual, 6–8 feet tall SACRED POWERS helps build confidence and courage; brings longevity

Fennel is in the carrot family and is edible, with flavors of anise or licorice. Its feathery leaves are commonly used as a garnish or spice, while its stalks are used raw or cooked in numerous recipes; it is also used in soaps, insect repellents, and dyes. Beneficial insects love the umbrella-shaped cluster of yellow flowers, which turns into tasty and fertile seeds that spread easily. The plant is well known for its anticancer and antioxidant properties and its ability to help with digestive and respiratory issues. In Chinese medicine, Xiao Hui Xiang (fennel seed and fennel fruit) is a warming herb used to alleviate colds and pain, and help the liver and kidneys. In Ayurvedic medicine, fennel is known as a cooling herb with benefits for the skin, digestion, heart, blood, and beauty, and to help with pain and as a fat buster when ingested as a tea. During the Middle Ages, fennel was hung in doorways to help ward off malevolent spirits.

FEVERFEW

Chrysanthemum parthenium

OTHER COMMON NAMES featherfew, wild chamomile GROWTH HABIT low and spreading, 2–3 feet tall SACRED POWERS rids a person of hexes, pain, and illness

This herbaceous perennial is a chamomile look-alike with very similar flowers, but the foliage is less fernlike and more leaflike. The aromatic properties are much different as well—chamomile is sweet compared to feverfew, which has more of a pungent smell. Feverfew leaves and flowers can be used fresh or dried in teas and tinctures to treat headaches and migraines, fever and inflammation, menstrual complaints, and circulation, and as a bitter tonic to help with digestion. To keep insects at bay, simply rub the leaves on your skin. Its essence helps ease nervous tension. During plague times, it was believed to help protect against disease if planted around one's house.

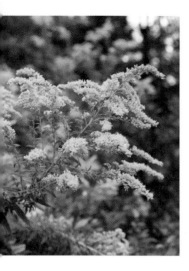

GOLDENROD

Solidago species

GROWTH HABIT sprawling or upright to 10 feet tall SACRED POWERS confers good luck and helps in the grieving process

The genus *Solidago* includes more than a hundred species, most native to North America. Goldenrod is not to be confused with the invasive ragweed whose pollen can cause severe allergies in some people, although the plants have similar yellow flowers that bloom at the same time. Goldenrod spreads underground through rhizomes, and its flowers attract many beneficial insects, including bees, butterflies, and wasps. The whole plant can be used, in tea, tinctures, and vinegars. The leaves are edible and can be used raw or dried. Medicinally, goldenrod has diuretic, astringent, antiseptic, antimicrobial, and anti-inflammatory properties helpful in healing the bladder and passing kidney stones. The tea can be used externally to treat skin injuries. Goldenrod also helps with respiratory illness, breaking up mucus and congestion. It can be used for dowsing, which simply means you hold a branch and ask to find something you are looking for; lore has it that it will nod in the direction of what you seek.

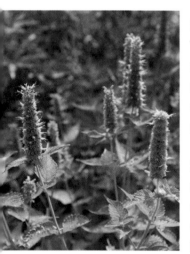

HYSSOP

Hyssopus officinalis

OTHER COMMON NAMES isopo, ysopo, yssop GROWTH HABIT upright stems to 2 feet tall SACRED POWERS offers purification and protection

In the mint family, this ancient herb has square stems, highly aromatic leaves, and flowers good for pollinators, as well as culinary, medicinal, and magical uses. In the kitchen, its fresh or dried leaves or flowers can be used to impart a strong minty flavor. Its medicinal uses include stimulating the gastrointestinal system, bringing up mucus from the lungs, and easing respiratory ailments; hyssop oil is used as an antiseptic. Hyssop is mentioned in the Bible as a purifier—"Thou shalt purge me with hyssop, and I shall be clean" (Psalms 51:7). This plant or water infused with it was used in ancient Greece and Egypt in rituals and ceremony to cleanse a sacred space. Bathing in it was believed to remove curses and to prevent the plague.

LADY'S MANTLE

Alchemilla mollis, A. vulgaris

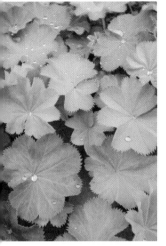

OTHER COMMON NAMES lion's foot, nine hooks, bear's foot GROWTH HABIT rounded, 1–2 feet tall and wide SACRED POWERS associated with goddess energy, including that of the Virgin Mary; enhances beauty when dew drops are gathered from the leaves and applied to the skin

Lady's mantle enjoys a shady spot in the garden, where it will spread into a nice ground cover. The enchanting leaves with nine lobes and finely cut edges delicately hold dew throughout the day. It blooms in the summer with frothy clusters of small yellow flowers. Lady's mantle has been used for centuries as a medicine; the whole plant—leaves, roots, and flowers—has astringent properties. It has been a remedy to treat issues relating to women's reproductive organs and tissues, such as relieving menstrual cramps and excessive menstrual bleeding. One source even claims it helps to restore or firm up saggy breast tissue. Studies have shown that lady's mantle tea can help with weight loss, is a powerful antioxidant, and helps lessen cough and flu symptoms.

LEMON BALM

Melissa officinalis

OTHER COMMON NAMES balm mint, garden balm, sweet balm, cure-all GROWTH HABIT upright, spreading, 2–3 feet tall SACRED POWERS sacred to the goddess Diana; symbolizes peace and purification; heals emotions and promotes longevity

Lemon balm is among my favorite "weeds" with its fragrant heart-shaped leaves. Its seeds have the ability to grow just about anywhere; to control its spread as an invasive, simply cut the flowers before they have a chance to go to seed. As a medicine, lemon balm is best known as an effective and gentle sedative, antiviral, and antibacterial. The volatile oils have been proven to be antispasmodic, soothing the overstimulated nervous system, anxiety, and insomnia. The leaves and flowers can be used fresh or dried in teas, tinctures, and ointments, but note that the plant's potency decreases significantly compared to other herbs once it is dried. This is my go-to plant when I'm feeling down—it instantly lifts my spirits yet is grounding at the same time.

MEADOWSWEET

Filipendula species

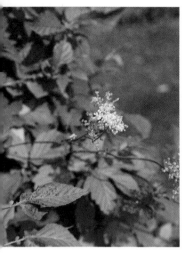

OTHER COMMON NAMES mead wort, meadow queen, meadsweet GROWTH HABIT erect stems to 4 feet tall SACRED POWERS symbolizes love and peace; helps heal emotional blocks from trauma such as fear and anger

This sweetly fragrant herb is often found in moist meadows with beautiful white plumes of summer-blooming flowers. The flowers are favored by bees and scented like almonds, while the leaves are more reminiscent of wintergreen. The whole plant is useful and historically was used to flavor wines and beers. Medicinally, meadowsweet has astringent and anti-inflammatory properties, and it contains salicylate (a natural aspirin). Meadowsweet is known to help with arthritis, general pain, and stomach complaints or digestive issues. It can reduce fevers and diarrhea in children. An herb sacred to Druids, the plant was traditionally used in love spells and as a strewing plant, spread on floors to impart fragrance to dwellings. Meadowsweet is used in bridal bouquets to symbolize a joyful, loving marriage.

MILKWEED

Asclepias species

GROWTH HABIT upright stalks 1–6 feet tall, spreading through rhizomes SACRED POWERS helps with self-reliance; balances neediness and emotional dependency

The genus *Asclepias* includes more than 150 species that grow in full sun and bloom in summer. Milkweed is a host plant for many insects and butterflies, making it a great addition to a wildlife garden. It is the only source of food for the larvae of the monarch butterfly, which has suffered a steep decline in population in recent years. The plant contains a milky sap that was once considered a good substitute for rubber, and it also contains compounds that repel some pests, so it is a useful companion plant. Some milkweed species were cooked and eaten as vegetables by Native Americans; they cannot be eaten raw, and some species are toxic. Many Native American tribes used the plants medicinally. The sap was used to remove warts and treat other skin ailments; a tonic from the roots was used to treat respiratory ailments. Even doctors prescribed the plant's medicine regularly in the 1800s. Herbalists still use some species for treating conditions of the lungs and detoxifying. The seed fluff, known as floss, absorbs oil but not water, making it useful as an insulation material and for oil spill cleanup.

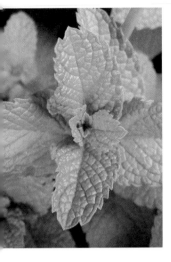

MINT

Mentha species

GROWTH HABIT spreading ground cover, 8–12 inches tall **SACRED POWERS** confers healing and protection

I consider mint the gateway plant to herbalism because it is so easy to grow. The genus *Mentha* includes many species and many, many hybrids and cultivars, including a chocolate and an apple mint. In general, this perennial herb is fast growing, enjoys rich and moist soils, and spreads by underground runners, giving it the ability to colonize garden beds quickly and become invasive. Pollinators love mint flowers, and the plant deters pesky insects like flies, so planting it in a container by the back door serves double duty. It is used in cosmetics and perfumes, as a natural pesticide, and as a culinary and medicinal herb. Fresh or dried mint leaves make a tea good for a variety of digestive system complaints, such as nausea, stomach ache, and gas, as well as for respiratory complaints and bad breath.

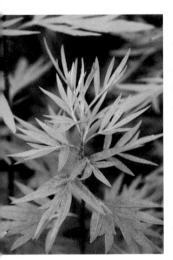

MUGWORT

Artemisia vulgaris

OTHER COMMON NAMES Artemis herb, cronewort, moxa **GROWTH HABIT** clumping, 4–6 feet tall **SACRED POWERS** protects travelers; induces lucid and prophetic dreams

Hands down, mugwort is my favorite plant to introduce women to. I remember the first time I met mugwort, at a Korean women's spa; there was a giant pool of water infused with mugwort to scoop out and pour all over our naked bodies. The plant's volatile oils have antifungal and antibacterial properties and thus enhance the cleansing effect of bathing rituals. Infusions of this plant can be used for cleaning around the house and as an insect repellent. The plant is edible and is often used in recipes for poultry stuffing; historically, it was used in beer. The leaves and flowers can be made into teas and tinctures; they can also be smoked and used as incense. Mugwort is one of the most ancient herbs, used in traditional medicine in China, India, Korea, and Europe. As a bitter it helps the digestive system and women's reproductive organs, although it should not be used during pregnancy. As an adjunct to acupuncture, dried mugwort is lit and held near certain points on the skin in a treatment known as moxibustion.

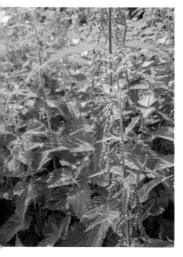

NETTLE

Urtica dioica

GROWTH HABIT erect spikes growing in dense clumps, 3–9 feet tall SACRED POWERS represents healing and protection; can be worn or planted to ward off negativity

Widely used in herbal medicine, nettle also offers an array of benefits as food, fiber, and soil conditioner. It grows in many parts of the world as an understory plant where there are rich and moist soils. The notable sting of nettle is from the fine hairs on the leaves, which inject chemical compounds when they are touched. Be sure to wear thick gloves and long sleeves when harvesting! Packed with important nutrients and minerals, this plant can be eaten as a cooked vegetable with a taste similar to spinach. As a medicine, the plant makes a detoxifying tonic that strengthens all body systems. It builds blood and helps improve resistance to environmental toxins such as pollutants, allergens, and molds. It can also be used as an astringent, diuretic, anti-inflamatory, antiseptic, and expectorant. Use fresh or dried leaves to make teas and tinctures, as well as oils, salves, and ointments for topical use. You can also make a green dye from the plant or use the tea as a hair rinse.

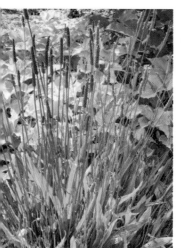

PLANTAIN

Plantago lanceolata, P. major, P. media

OTHER COMMON NAMES ripple grass, waybread, snakeweed, cuckoo's bread, Englishman's foot, white man's foot GROWTH HABIT upright stems, 8–12 inches tall SACRED POWERS symbolizes strength, healing, and protection—especially from snakes

Plantago species number in the couple of hundreds and are found all over the world, growing in abundance in a variety of habitats. Several of these species are perennial "weeds" that are valuable and accessible medicinal plants. The shape of the leaf depends on the species, but all have deep ribs that are edible—if bitter—when young, and all have flowers on tall stalks. Medicinally, plantain has been used since prehistoric times, and the plant is still used fresh in teas, tinctures, and infused oils as a salve or ointment. The fresh leaves can be mashed or bruised to use topically as a poultice or made into a compress to heal skin irritations like rashes, cuts, and insect bites, and to draw out toxins from poisonous insects. Plantain is diuretic, astringent, anti-inflammatory, antimicrobial, and mucilaginous, and can heal respiratory irritations, mouth issues, and tooth pain.

Native Americans called plantain white man's foot because wherever European settlers went, the plant followed.

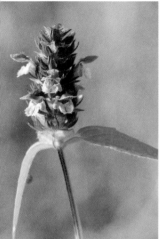

SELF-HEAL
Prunella vulgaris

OTHER COMMON NAMES heal-all, woundwort GROWTH HABIT spreading ground cover, 12–18 inches tall SACRED POWERS assists with working magic if harvested at night, in the dark of the moon, and placed on an altar

Self-heal is a low-growing, creeping perennial ground cover with purplish blue flowers on short stalks. It grows throughout temperate climates as a common weed in gardens, on ecosystem edges, and in disturbed areas, and prefers moist, rich soils. The leaves and flowers are edible raw or cooked and can be used fresh or dried to make teas and tinctures. Dried

into a powder, self-heal can be used in beverages. The astringent plant has many constituents that make it an excellent wound healer, and it is being studied in western medicine for its antibiotic and antioxidant properties. The plant's antiviral properties make it a useful remedy for the flu, sore throats, and cold sores. Made into a salve, it can be kept in your first aid kit and used topically for skin issues. In Chinese medicine, self-heal is known as Xia Ku Cao and is considered a cooling bitter medicine good for removing heat, protecting the liver, and improving eyesight.

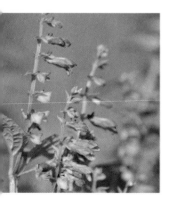

SKULLCAP
Scutellaria lateriflora

OTHER COMMON NAMES hoodwort, helmet flower, mad dog skullcap GROWTH HABIT upright spikes, 1–4 feet tall SACRED POWERS promotes love, fidelity, and peace

Its miniature helmetlike blue flowers give this perennial mint its common name.

Many species grow throughout the world in temperate climates, but not all are interchangeable. *Scutellaria lateriflora* is a North American native that prefers moist soils and grows well in the shade as an understory plant. It is an important nervine in western herbalism, a great natural sedative that helps calm anxiety and restore a frayed nervous system. It can help with insomnia and promote restful sleep. It is also anti-inflammatory, antispasmodic, slightly astringent, and a tonic. It is used to treat pain and depression as well as drug addiction withdrawal symptoms. The leaves and flowers can be used fresh or dried in teas and tinctures or in powdered capsule form. In Chinese medicine, the root of *Scutellaria baicalensis*, Huang Qin, is one of the fundamental herbs, a cold bitter that helps clear heat and dry dampness.

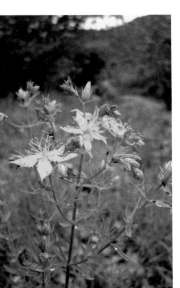

ST. JOHN'S WORT　　　　*Hypericum perforatum*

OTHER COMMON NAMES goat weed, herba John, St. Joan's wort GROWTH HABIT spreading ground cover up to 2 feet tall SACRED POWERS used to protect against and ward off evil spirits and ill health; attracts love and is associated with nature spirits

St. John's wort is native to Europe and was used as a medicine as early as the first century AD in Greece. The flower makes a nice yellow dye, and the plant's roots create a dense ground cover, making it effective for erosion control or as a living mulch. However, as an ornamental ground cover it can also become an aggressive weed in many gardens, often taking over in spaces where the plant is happy. It can also be toxic to livestock when eaten in sufficient quantity. Medicinally, it has a long list of healing properties, including being an antidepressant, an anti-inflammatory, a liver detoxifier, an antibiotic for first aid, and a treatment for nerve damage. Magically, it was believed to ward off evil spirits if hung in the entrance to a building, placed in a jar, worn, or burned. Placing it under one's pillow was believed to cause dreams of future love. It is used in midsummer rituals—burned, made into garlands, and infused into oils for anointing. A cautionary note: it can alter the effectiveness of certain medications, including birth control, and should not be used during breastfeeding or pregnancy.

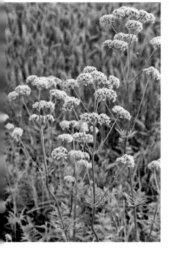

VALERIAN

Valeriana officinalis

OTHER COMMON NAMES all-heal, capon's tail, garden heliotrope, setwall, vandal root GROWTH HABIT clumping, with erect stems up to 6 feet tall SACRED POWERS performs dream magic; symbolizes peace, harmony, and love; confers protection

This perennial herb is native to Europe and Asia, and was mentioned by Hippocrates, who noted its roots' effectiveness as a medicine. It was also once used as a spice and perfume but is best known as a relaxant, calming the nervous system and muscles, helping with tension or sleeplessness. Valerian has strong sedative effects and can be used at times of intense anxiety or stress but should not be used with other depressants. The dried root smells somewhat like a stinky sock, and I recommend taking honey with your tea if you use it that way. The fresh root can also be used in a tincture or a bath. Traditionally used in Samhain (Halloween) and Yule rituals, the herb has also had many magical uses, including casting love spells and protecting from evil and nightmares.

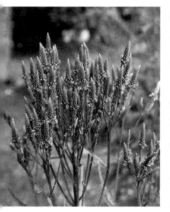

VERVAIN

Verbena hastata, V. officinalis

OTHER COMMON NAMES verbena, herb of the cross, Indian hyssop GROWTH HABIT erect stems to 3–5 feet tall SACRED POWERS helps with balance and centering, with releasing and clearing, and with divination

Verbena hastata and *V. officinalis* are drought-tolerant perennials with flowers that are usually blue but can be purple, pink, or white. Pollinators and butterflies love the flowers, making vervain a great plant for wildlife habitat. Medicinally, it has traditionally been used as a digestive bitter, to treat kidney stones, and to help alleviate depression and anxiety. Many Native American tribes used *V. hastata* as a tonic for a number of ailments, including breast complaints, colds, cough, digestive complaints, and fevers. Its history as a sacred plant spans the ages; in ancient Egypt, it was known as the plant that comes from the tears of the goddess Isis, while the ancient Greeks and Romans referred to it as the holy plant and used it to clean altars. It is also thought to have been the herb that dressed Jesus' wounds when he was taken down from the cross. In the magical realm, it is used in potions and spells to heal a broken heart, for good luck, and to lighten a dark mood, among other things.

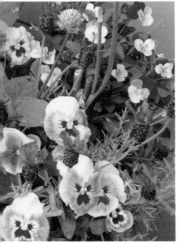

VIOLET

Viola odorata

OTHER COMMON NAMES sweet violet, wild pansy GROWTH HABIT creeping, mounding, 2–10 inches tall SACRED POWERS symbolizes protection, lust, and peace; brings good luck or healing after a painful breakup or loss

This sweet little flower often marks the beginning of springtime. It is often thought of interchangeably with *Viola tricolor* (Johnny jump-up, heartsease) but *V. tricolor* usually has three colors instead of one or two, and *V. odorata* is especially fragrant and used as an ingredient in perfume or cosmetics. Both have been adored for thousands of years, used in folk medicine and cuisine. Medicinally, both have anti-inflammatory, diuretic, and expectorant properties. Both are used for respiratory illnesses like bronchitis and coughs, and are also applied topically for skin ailments. Violets are easy to use in herbal teas and tinctures. *Viola odorata* was a symbol of love in ancient Greece and was thought to calm anger when worn.

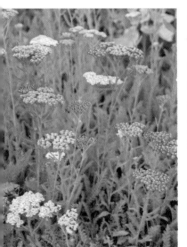

YARROW

Achillea millefolium

OTHER COMMON NAMES millfoil, devil's nettle, soldier's woundwort GROWTH HABIT upright stalks to 3 feet tall SACRED POWERS in dream pillows, brings prophetic dreams; useful in love spells

This hardy perennial has made its way around the globe and has been carbon dated at sixty thousand years old. The plant has fernlike foliage and tall stalks topped with clusters of dainty flowers in many hues. As it grows just about anywhere, is drought tolerant, and spreads easily by seed, yarrow is commonly found in lawns, along roadways, and in cultivated gardens. Ecologically, it provides nectar for pollinators and beneficial insects. The young leaves and flowers are edible and can be used in salads. The fresh leaves can be chewed to relieve toothache or applied to the skin to stop bleeding; for centuries, soldiers used to carry dried yarrow leaves into battle to treat wounds. Made into a salve, yarrow has anti-inflammatory properties and soothes arthritis. To make an insect repellent, simply make an infusion. Yarrow is also known to help strengthen properties of other plants when used in combinations.

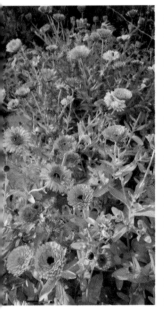

CALENDULA   *Calendula officinalis*

OTHER COMMON NAMES desert marigold, pot marigold GROWTH HABIT clumping, 1–3 feet tall and wide SACRED POWERS brings comfort to the heart

This cheery annual blooms throughout the summer into late fall and is an excellent edible, medicinal, and dye plant. It looks beautiful as a garnish on salads and soups, and is also a favorite of pollinators. Calendula is easy to grow and reseeds itself, making a good naturalizing ground cover. Studies have shown that the plant has anti-inflammatory, antiviral, and antigenotoxic properties and can treat a variety of skin ailments as well as problems with digestion and women's issues. The plant is used in Chinese and Ayurvedic medicine and by Native Americans for similar treatments. The flowers can be used to make teas, tinctures, and infused oils, which can then be used in salves and ointments. Calendula was used in ceremonies and rituals in ancient Greece and Rome and has been considered sacred in India.

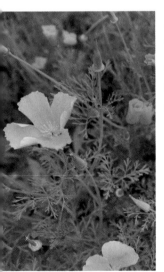

CALIFORNIA POPPY   *Eschscholzia californica*

OTHER COMMON NAMES golden poppy GROWTH HABIT 4–12 inches tall and wide SACRED POWERS represents sleep, and the peace of the dead; calms without becoming addictive

Known to some gardeners as a weed, this powerful plant self-sows easily, as an annual in colder climates, spreading to just about any soil left disturbed in the sun. It is great for those areas hard to grow in—dry, difficult soils. It blooms throughout the summer until frost, with cultivars available in different colors, though the offspring are likely to grow back to orange. The flowers, leaves, and seeds are all useful for quieting insomnia and also for quelling anxiety or stress. With its mild sedative effect, California poppy is gentle and safe for adults and children, without the same addictive properties as its relative opiate poppy. It can be used as a tea or tincture and is a bitter good for digestion. Native American tribes have used this plant in pain relief remedies for headaches and toothaches, and in poultices. It has been said to work well as a hair tonic and to help with addictions and drug abuse.

CHAMOMILE

Matricaria recutita (German chamomile), *Chamaemelum nobile* (Roman chamomile)

OTHER COMMON NAMES mayweed, ground apple, earth apple GROWTH HABIT German, annual, 2 feet tall; Roman, perennial, 6–12 inches tall SACRED POWERS helps with improving luck, attracting love, and creating peace

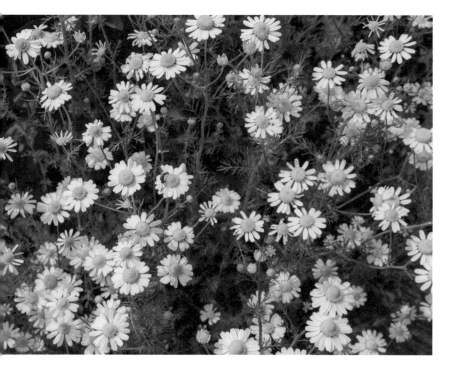

Several different plants are known as chamomile. All have small white daisylike flowers, and two species are distinctly well known for their medicinal value. Roman chamomile has petals facing downward, smells like apple, and makes a great ground cover. German chamomile grows taller and has feathery foliage. Both grow in sunny areas and can tolerate poor soils. Chamomile is known medically for its anti-inflammatory, antibacterial, antifungal, and sedative properties, and has been used for centuries as a cure-all tonic. The bitters have been proven to help with the digestive tract and a number of women's issues. It also makes a great hair rinse for blond hair. In folk medicine, chamomile was considered the remedy for babies, helping to gently treat colic, teething, gas, and insomnia. In Chinese medicine, chamomile is known to help with tension and heat, toning the liver and moving qi energy. Its essence helps ease emotional tension, bringing a sunny disposition.

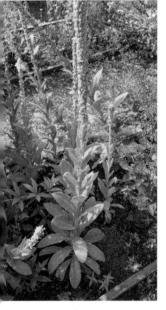

MULLEIN   *Verbascum* species

OTHER COMMON NAMES velvet dock, candle-wick plant, beggar's blanket, old man's flannel **GROWTH HABIT** central stalk, 3–5 feet tall **SACRED POWERS** symbolizes courage, strength, and divination; offers protection when worn in shoes or carried in sachets

This biennial grows with a large rosette of fuzzy leaves giving rise to a stalk with yellow flowers in summer. It grows just about anywhere and is most commonly found at the edges of disturbed areas. It hosts many insects, both beneficial and

pests. Medicinally, mullein has been used for centuries as an emollient, demulcent, and astringent to treat illnesses and irritations of the respiratory system and skin. The leaves and flowers can be used fresh or dried, although the leaves can take time to dry thoroughly. In folk medicine, smoking the leaves was used as a remedy for coughs and asthma. Oil infusions can be useful for skin ailments and earaches. In dream pillows, mullein makes a soft filler material and protects from nightmares.

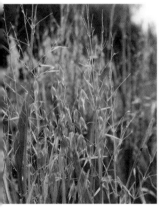

OAT   *Avena sativa*

OTHER COMMON NAMES oat seed, milkseed, oat straw **GROWTH HABIT** erect, 1–4 feet tall **SACRED POWERS** draws prosperity and money; helps with finding one's true path

Oat is an annual grass plant that has been grown as a staple grain for thousands of years. It is very common in the European diet and is also used medicinally. As a crop, it requires nitrogen-rich soils and is ideally rotated with a legume crop. Oats are rich in fiber, protein, vitamins, and minerals, benefiting the brain, heart, sex drive, nervous system, and skin.

As a nervine, oat helps restore the nervous system when one is stressed, aids relaxation, and can help relieve depression. Topically, it can soothe irritated or inflamed skin, and it is one of my favorite plants to use in a bath mix for soaking. Oat seeds are best used fresh in tinctures, or dried for later use in teas. The seeds are most edible when dried and processed. The whole plant, known as oat straw, can be harvested and dried for medicinal use.

QUEEN ANNE'S LACE   *Daucus carota*

OTHER COMMON NAMES wild carrot, bird's nest GROWTH HABIT erect, 1–4 feet tall SACRED POWERS enhances psychic ability, gives spiritual clarity, and aids fertility even though it prevents conception; in dream pillows, brings intuitive dreaming

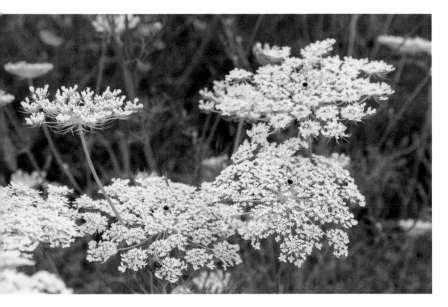

Queen Anne's lace, with its distinctive flat lacy cluster of white flowers, is often seen blooming along roadways in late summer but can also be cultivated in a wildflower garden. This biennial is host to many beneficial insects—in particular wasps, lacewings, ladybugs, hoverflies, and bees. The young root is edible and diuretic, and the seeds and oils have been used for a number of ailments including colic, kidney stones, parasites, and flatulence. Queen Anne's lace has also been used as a natural contraceptive since the fifth century and is being studied for a number of other treatments. Brew a decoction and use the antiseptic and astringent tonic for cleansing your skin. *Caution*—this plant looks very similar to water hemlock, which is highly poisonous. Water hemlock has a smooth stem while Queen Anne has "hairy legs."

RED CLOVER   *Trifolium pratense*

GROWTH HABIT clumping, 6–24 inches tall and wide SACRED POWERS offers protection and good luck

Biennial red clover is a weed to gardeners, a protein-rich fodder to farmers, and a versatile medicine to herbalists.

Ecologically, it makes an ideal cover crop as it fixes nitrogen and enriches soils. It is also an important nectar source for pollinators, which it depends on for fertilization. Medicinally, the plant has been used for centuries around the world to treat a wide array of ailments. Red clover is known as an expectorant useful in treating respiratory issues like bronchitis, cough, and asthma, and is also well known for helping women with PMS and postmenopause symptoms. It is an edible nutritive and blood purifier, making a good detoxifying tonic, and is used topically to treat skin problems in children. It has even been proven in studies to act as an antibiotic to the pathogen that causes tuberculosis and is being studied for its role in treating cancer.

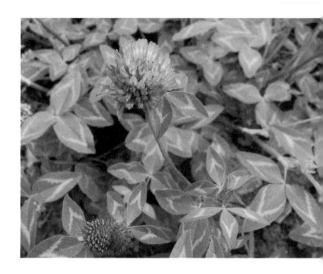

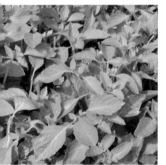

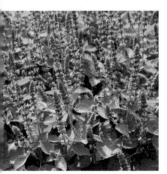

TULSI

Ocimum tenuiflorum

OTHER COMMON NAMES holy basil, sacred basil, surasa, tulasi GROWTH HABIT upright, 2 feet tall and wide SACRED POWERS promotes longevity

Known as the queen of herbs, tulsi has a rich several-thousand-year history and powerful strengths as a healer. It grows as an annual in temperate climates, as a perennial in tropical and subtropical ones. Related to culinary basil, it loves sun and does well in neutral soils, attracting bees and pollinators. Its constituents have antibacterial, antidepressant, antioxidant, antiviral, and expectorant properties. Tulsi helps with colds and respiratory ailments, memory, oral care, wound care, stress relief, kidney care, and headaches; it also protects from heart disease and prevents premature aging. In Eastern medicine, it is used to support normal cortisol and blood sugar levels. Ayurvedic medicine considers it a warm bitter, good to clear mental fog and keep the chakras balanced. It is easiest to benefit from as a tea; drink it daily, perhaps as a coffee substitute, to notice a difference in your health. In Hinduism, tulsi is considered a sacred plant and placed on altars, made into prayer beads, and used in ceremony. Ancient folklore holds it to be the manifestation of the divine mother on earth.

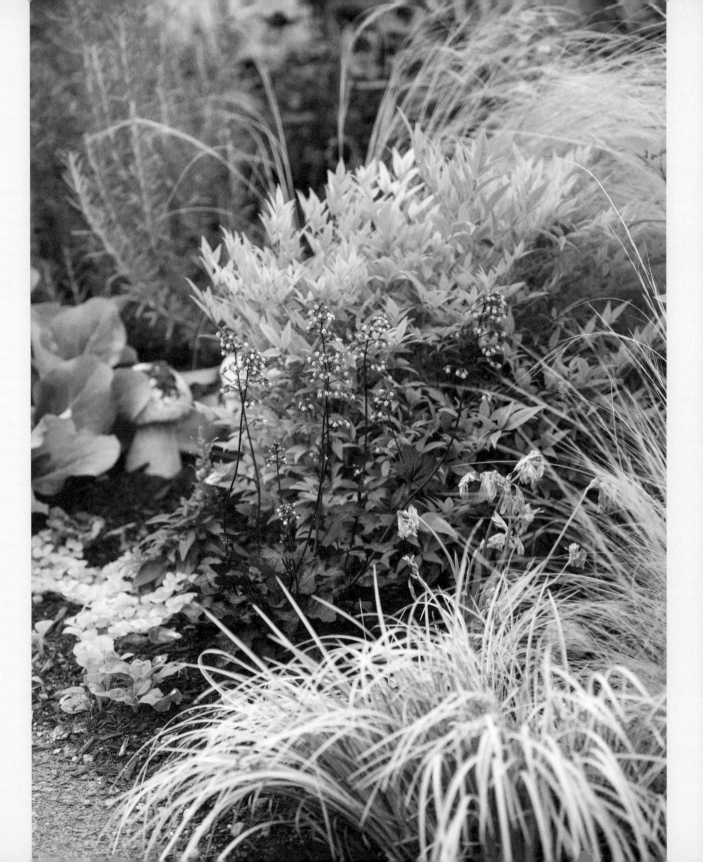

Plant Spirit Medicine

PLANTS AS OUR ALLIES

Plant allies come in all shapes and sizes, and we can carefully choose which ones to include in our sanctuary.

Plants are incredible healers. They can provide support to us in every aspect of our day-to-day lives if we know how to use them. They can aid us with our emotional states, our relationships, and our spiritual consciousness. If we start to tune in to the vital life force energy plants provide, we can use their power to help us achieve wellness of body, spirit, and mind. The key is to begin looking at plants as our allies.

Throughout every day of my life, I ask myself which plant can help me out. If I wake up on the wrong side of the bed or get stressed from raising my kids or from work deadlines, there is a plant to help. If I have a stomachache or feel sad, I know some plants that can help with that. If my body is tired or my mind is racing, there are plants for that.

If you want to feel different, plants can help you get to where you want to go. Your sacred space will be both more meaningful and more useful if you develop a relationship with each species of plant you intend to grow and use. Beyond that, some knowledge of the healing properties of plants can help you decide which plant allies you want to include in your sanctuary and the specific uses you want to make of them.

Developing a Relationship with Your Plants

I often relate to plants as I do to people—building symbiotic and empathetic relationships. To do this, become familiar with your plants on an intimate level from the moment you meet them in the container at the nursery or watch your first seedling sprout, stretch its first baby leaf open, and reach for sunlight. To learn from your plants, watch them carefully and discover what they need from you. Learn to notice when a plant becomes thirsty and is asking for water. You

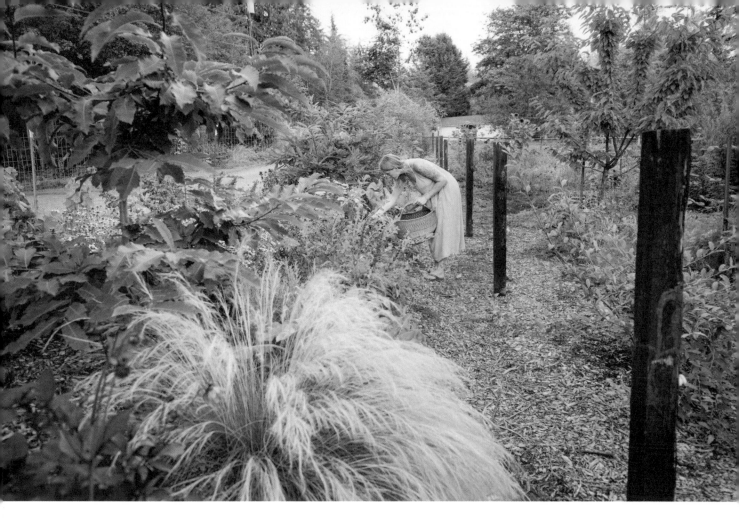

Building relationships with plants starts with tending and nurturing them.

become responsible for these plants as they grow into maturity. As you learn how to feed them, wean them, stake them, and prune them, you develop empathy with these silent little beings that require your care and nurturing.

Until you have really seen a plant grow from seed to flower to seed again, until you have used its medicine, until you have drunk from its leaves or bathed with its flower, you don't really know it as well as you could. Once you work with

elderly plants, you start to learn how much stress they can handle and nurture them as they age. You help defend them against pests and disease, you learn to prune out the dead limbs—or as I see it sometimes, comb their hair. Until you have tended a plant throughout its reproductive cycle, you may not fully appreciate what it has to offer and how it can help you. With each species that I have built a relationship with, I've been amazed at the depth of the continual

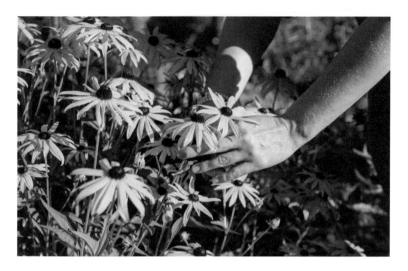

When you have a relationship with a plant, you pay attention to its health throughout its life cycle and consider its health when harvesting.

learning it can offer. And the more I learn, the more I realize I don't know.

I encourage you to consider these questions as you research which plants to have a relationship with and grow in your sanctuary:

* Plant behavior. What are the basics of the plant's genetic makeup? How big does it want to get? What are its likes and dislikes in terms of sun, shade, soil types, watering? Is the plant aggressive or passive, and how can you control it if it does become invasive?

* Ecological attributes. What purpose does the plant serve ecologically? Is it an early successional species or pioneer? What can it do for people and other organisms or as an ecological function? Plants can have specific niches such as pollinator food source, soil builder, or habitat structural element.

* Plant spirit or energy. What is this plant's story? Historically, what did the plant offer the human psyche? What did it symbolize? What is the folklore or mythology or traditional spiritual healing use associated with this plant? What are the well-known uses of the plant?

Once you start thinking in these terms about each plant you might place in your sanctuary space, you will already be expanding your sense of the help available to you there.

I would suggest that you connect with the plants you are most familiar with first. Which plants do you remember fondly from your childhood or already have a relationship with? Using plants that currently grow in your garden or bioregion is a great place to start. Then you can learn plants from your heritage or genetic lineage, from the regions where your ancestors lived. Spend time in stillness and full presence close to your chosen plants and open yourself to exchanging energy with them.

The Wisdom of Weeds

Eeyore in *Winnie the Pooh* said, "Weeds are flowers too, once you get to know them." I've always thought that the weeds we encounter have much to teach us. They are wonderful models of persistence and patience. They are good indicators

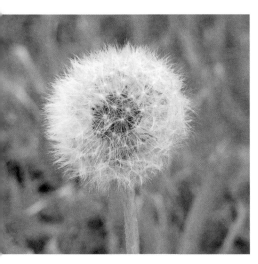

Dandelion, usually considered a weed, contains potent life force energy that can be used for healing.

of what is happening in the soil. Like nature's repair crew, they prevent soil loss, produce biomass, and improve fertility in disturbed soils. One of the main ecological services of weeds is simply to cover the ground and prepare the soil for the next plant community in succession. Besides, weeds can be nutritionally dense foods—and easy to grow! And many weeds are safe, potent medicines that can help us heal our bodies.

Yet often, people can get overwhelmed with weeds and weeding. This can take away from the joy and feeling of sanctuary the garden can offer. But do you really need to worry about controlling them? Every climate has its "problem" plants—and some weed species can be an asset in your garden. For instance, dandelion is rich in minerals and nutrients, and is often found in soil where calcium is needed. Clover, a nitrogen-fixing plant, often shows up when the soil is nitrogen deficient and remedies the problem. Knowing that exposed soil will continually produce vegetation until another species takes over, you can plant with the intention of covering every inch of bare soil so that weeds will have no space to flourish. You can also consider weeds a gift and harvest them for their nutritional and medicinal uses. Following

are descriptions of six common weeds that are useful if you know what to do with them.

Burdock, *Arctium lappa*, *A. minor*
Burdock—also known as thorny burr, beggar's buttons, lappa, or gypsy rhubarb—is a weed common in many parts of the world. It is most remembered for its seeds or burrs, which were the inspiration for Velcro and which travel to new ground attached to fur and clothing like a little hitchhiker. It grows in hedgerows, along roadsides, and at the edges of ecosystems, with big, fleshy, wavy leaves, developing a deep taproot system. Burdock root has been used medicinally to cleanse blood, the liver, and the skin. You can dig burdock roots for fresh use or dry them and make a tincture or other extracts. The leaves make a great poultice for skin irritations; just steam the leaves and put on skin for twenty minutes. Spiritually, burdock helps cleanse negative feelings held toward the self.

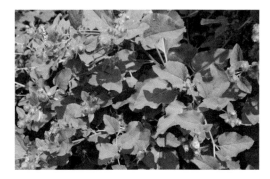

Burdock, *Arctium lappa*

Chickweed, *Stellaria media* This herbaceous annual grows around the world, easily naturalizing, with small white star-shaped flowers on trailing and often tangled succulent branches. It is a common weed to some, and an edible and medicinal plant to others. Typically

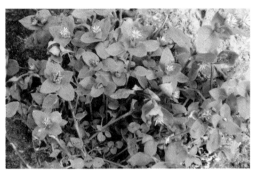

Chickweed, *Stellaria media*

you can find it in moist and shady parts of the garden or on the edges of ecosystems in the cooler seasons. Full of minerals, nutrients, and vitamins (A, B1, B2, B6, B12, C), this plant is known as a spring vegetable good for digestion. It is edible either raw or cooked and makes an excellent base for a salad or in sandwiches. You can make a tincture to have on hand when the plant is not in season; though not as nutritious as the whole plant parts, this tincture can help the kidneys regulate water internally, which has made chickweed known as an obesity remedy that helps to reduce water weight. Fresh or dried, it can be infused into a tea. It is a cooling and moist herb, great at helping with skin irritations such as burns, wounds, and insect bites. Make a poultice from fresh leaves, or dry the plant and make infused oil, which can be applied externally or made into a healing salve. Spiritually, chickweed teaches humility and flexibility; it helps with

fertility as well as maintaining relationships by cooling our anger.

Dandelion, *Taraxacum officinale*
Perhaps the most widely recognized plant, dandelion is known as food and used as medicine around the world—yet in the garden and lawn industry, it is regarded as an unwelcome weed that develops a deep taproot and spreads seeds easily. Ecologically, as a pioneer species it helps develop soil on disturbed sites, especially in compacted sunny areas, bringing nutrients and minerals to

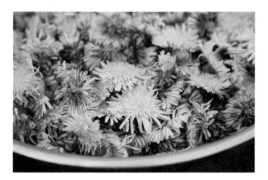

Dandelion, *Taraxacum officinale*

the surface and breaking up the soil. It is a source of food and pollen for beneficial insects and other critters. The whole plant is useful: the leaves are an edible bitter green, the petals have been used in beverages such as beer and wine, and the root is used in teas or even as a caffeine-free coffee substitute. Medicinally, dandelions have been used in many cultures for centuries for their detoxifying effects.

Dandelion is used in teas as a detoxifying tonic, as a diuretic, and as an aid to liver function and digestion. Its sacred powers include granting wishes when the seed heads are blown on and calling in spirits when boiling water is poured over a bowl full of roots.

_____

Dock, *Rumex crispus* Dock is a strong and humble weed commonly found

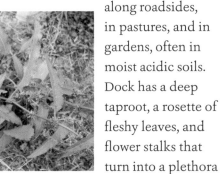

Dock, *Rumex crispus*

along roadsides, in pastures, and in gardens, often in moist acidic soils. Dock has a deep taproot, a rosette of fleshy leaves, and flower stalks that turn into a plethora of unique three-sided seeds that easily colonize an area. The plant is food for butterfly larvae. Yellow dock is the species best known as a useful herb to treat a variety of ailments. The young leaves can be eaten and taste astringent and slightly sour; with age, the leaves become less palatable due to oxalic acid building in the tissues. Growing conditions may also affect flavor. The seeds can be ground into flour or used as a garnish. The roots can be used raw or dried and made into teas, decoctions, tinctures, and salves. The herb is used to treat skin ailments, as a laxative, for digestive issues, and to cleanse the blood and remove toxins. Among its

sacred powers, dock brings good luck, helps to clean up old emotional baggage, and increases fertility.

_____

Lamb's quarters, *Chenopodium album* This annual plant grows throughout the world and is a useful superfood, ecological ally, and medicinal. It grows in a variety of conditions, from waste sites to cultivated gardens, but favors rich soils and can be an indicator of good soil health. It is helpful to farmers and gardeners as a companion plant for its ability to attract leaf miners away from other plants. It is a nutritional food source for chickens, other poultry, and livestock. The spring greens are full of nutrients and minerals, and especially high in vitamin C, along with providing vitamin A and the B complex. The seeds are also edible and high in protein. Medicinally, the herb is an astringent, anti-inflammatory, and laxative. It can be chewed and applied directly to the skin as a poultice

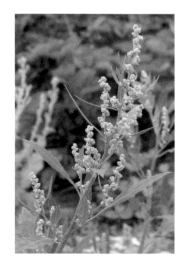

Lamb's quarters, *Chenopodium album*

for minor irritations like insect stings, bites, and sunburns. As a tea it can be used externally to treat ailments or in the bath to tone the skin. It can also be taken internally for digestive issues and as a detox tonic. The roots contain saponin, an ingredient of soap, and can be used in bathing or in a hair rinse.

Purslane, *Portulaca oleracea* This herbaceous annual has small succulent leaves and spreads horizontally. Ecologically, it holds moisture close to the soil and is thus a helpful companion plant to others that need moisture. Purslane contains nutrients, minerals, and more omega-3 fatty acids than any other plant and is considered one of the healthiest vegetables we can eat. It is used throughout the world raw or cooked in soups, salads, and even pastries, although it should not be eaten during pregnancy. The plant tissues can be squeezed to make a juice to drink or use topically, and the pulp has hydrating and toning properties and is an ingredient in beauty care and bathing products. As a medicine, purslane is anti-inflamatory, antibacterial, and diuretic, and is easily made into poultices or cold compresses. Among its sacred powers, it induces peaceful sleep, confers protection during travel, and works as a love charm and for good luck.

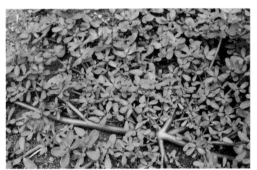

Purslane, *Portulaca oleracea*

Earth-Based Healing and Traditional Medicine

The more I study plants, the more fascinated I am with not only the biological details but also the history of each plant's use throughout human civilization. Ethnobotany, the study of humans' historical relationships to plants, can be a valuable tool when learning about how we might use plants today. It reveals that many different cultures, religions, and belief systems have used plants—for a multitude of purposes—all the way back to the beginnings of human civilization. Everywhere in the world, the use of plants was essential for survival of the first peoples. Plants provided food, medicine, clothing, shelter, tools, and spiritual practice, and that wisdom was shared collectively and often passed down as oral tradition.

Some plants have been used to help expand human consciousness, to enhance levels of perception and thinking. These visionary plants are considered teachers with the ability to communicate nature's wisdom. Such plants as peyote, ayahuasca, marijuana, poppy, and psilocybin mushrooms have psychoactive properties and were traditionally used to nourish the psyche and soul with the aid of a guide during ceremony. Some of these plants—or fungi—are now being used in modern psychological practices for healing mental illnesses. Psilocybin is used as a substitute for antidepressants in what is called microdosing—giving a small, regular dose of the substance.

Originally, medicines came from the earth. Medicine women and men had intimate experience and relationships with local plants and could pair ailing people with the right ones for healing. Knowledge of a plant's healing potency was passed from generation to generation in pre-industrial societies around the globe. This knowledge was obtained by lots of trial and error, from observing other species' use of plants, and from spiritual teachings. Many pharmaceuticals we use today that are synthesized in a laboratory originated as plant derivatives (also known as biopiracy), although it might be hard to find out which of our prescriptions or supplements originally came from a plant's compounds. Natural medicines were pushed aside once pharmaceuticals came on the scene. Even though it has a much longer history than western medicine, herbal medicine in our society is touted as "alternative."

Shamanism, a belief system that dates back seventy thousand to one hundred thousand years, is chief among earth-based healing practices that makes use of herbs and herbal medicines. It has been present in nearly all human cultures around the planet, so it is safe to say that every modern human has ancestors who experienced shamanism. The underlying principle of this ancient practice is that all life has spirit and that we can choose to engage with this life energy and learn from it. The word *shaman* refers to someone (male or female) who has a deep relationship with the spirit world. A shaman can take many forms, and healing modalities vary with each practitioner but are based in earth healing.

Eastern medicine—particularly traditional Chinese medicine (TCM) and Ayurvedic medicine—also has a very long history and has relied on traditional knowledge of the healing properties of plants. Both TCM and Ayurveda look to the energy centers in our bodies for indications of wellness, and both use plants as aids in the process of healing.

Practiced for three thousand years, TCM was first rooted in Taoism. One of its core tenets is that chi (or qi, pronounced "chee"), the body's life force energy, moves through meridians and channels in the body. To maintain health, our bodies need a free flow of this energy. Blockages and disharmony cause disease. TCM treats and prevents health problems by guiding the body back to its natural state of balance through the use of herbal medicine, acupuncture, diet therapy, massage techniques, moxibustion (burning plant material on or near the surface of the skin), and tai chi and qigong (movement).

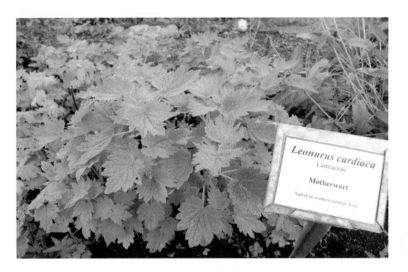

Traditional Chinese medicine has long made use of motherwort to promote longevity and treat menstrual disorders.

Ayurveda means "the science of life" and refers to an ancient holistic healing system that developed in India. Ayurveda first looks at our unique make-up or energetic constitution, which includes physical characteristics like skin, hair, and bone structure and also how we use our energy and emotions. The system defines three mind-body types or doshas—called vata, pitta, and kapha—and posits that each of us is made up of some unique combination of the three constitutions. Health is seen as a state of balance achieved when we are in living in tune with our inborn constitution and nature's cycles. Plants are also seen as having an energetic makeup, consisting of their taste, heaviness/lightness, heating/cooling, and digestive effects. Ayurvedic medicine connects us to plants and practices for wellness based on our constitution.

All of these systems point to the fact that plants can be powerful allies in our quest for health and well-being. In these healing systems and in other forms of traditional, indigenous, or folk medicine, plants' healing constituents are used in teas, foods and spices, tinctures, poultices, and smudge sticks. Their oils are used in aromatherapy, and their essences are used in preparations such as the Bach flower remedies (developed by Edward Bach in the 1930s in England). You can choose plants to include in your sanctuary garden that you can make use of for their healing properties. In the section that follows, you will find many suggestions about plants to use as allies to help with a variety of emotional/mental conditions.

Plants for Emotional Healing and Mental Well-Being

Medical systems and herbalism offer many resources to help heal physical ailments, but our culture doesn't always have systems set up to support us when we are not feeling well emotionally. Many rely on pharmaceuticals to treat symptoms when struggling with mental health or spiritual well-being. In creating sanctuary, it is important to think about nurturing our inner being. This means looking holistically at what we are dealing with inside. When we can face our emotional state, rather than masking the symptoms, it becomes easier to treat. Plants can aid us in this process, and we may also need

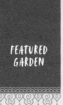
BASTYR UNIVERSITY HERBAL MEDICINE GARDEN

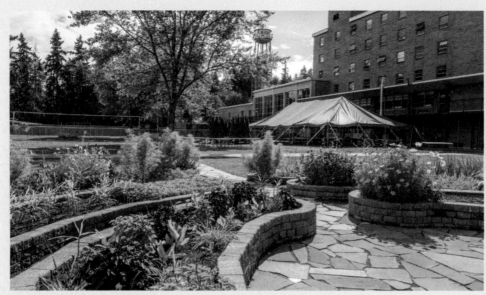

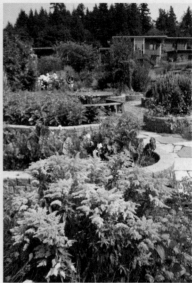

A central area contains raised beds in the botanical garden at Bastyr University.

ABOVE RIGHT The gardens at Bastyr are organized by uses—some medicinal and some ecological.

BASTYR UNIVERSITY, which opened in 1978, is regarded as one of the best colleges in the world teaching science-based natural medicine. Courses of study include naturopathy, Ayurvedic science, psychology, and nutrition. The 51-acre site northeast of Seattle where the school moved in 1996 was originally the home of a Catholic seminary, complete with an elegant European-style chapel adorned with glass art mosaics, marble columns, and tall arched ceilings creating a perfectly tuned venue for a variety of events. The grounds encompass large outdoor classrooms with demonstration medicinal gardens containing hundreds of plant allies, a reflexology foot path, and a sacred seed ethnobotany trail that illustrates historical uses of native plants as food and medicine and in ceremony.

The school is blessed in many ways, as are all who visit it. Each of the times I've been invited to teach at Bastyr has been a magical experience. I have felt surrounded by the spirit of the plants and the land, as well as of the humans who have so diligently dedicated their lives to learn about the healing properties of plants so they could share that wisdom to make humans healthy. By becoming the first naturopathic college to gain accreditation, Bastyr has led the way in creating a resurgence of interest in natural and plant-based medicine.

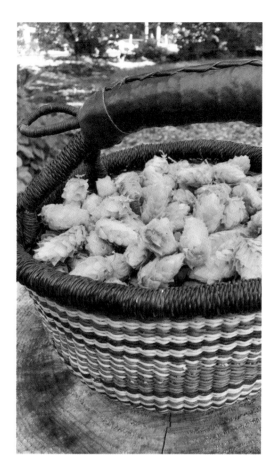

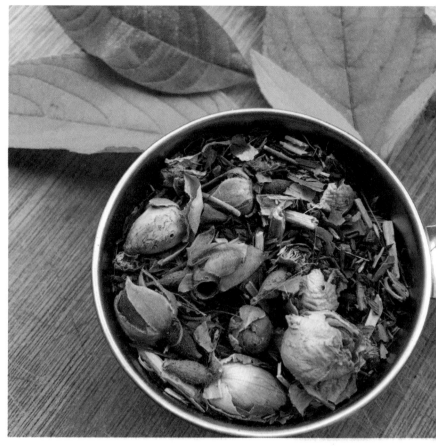

Plants such as these freshly harvested hops can help us maintain mental and emotional health.

ABOVE RIGHT One way to experiment with plants for health and healing is to start with existing blends of plant parts in teas and see what the effects are.

support from therapists, doctors, healers, and community.

Not everyone needs to become a credentialed herbalist or to master natural medicine to experiment with plants for health and healing. You can start by trying existing blends of plant parts in teas and see what the effects are for you. You may find that one plant does not work at all for you, while another plant works wonders. There are many things to learn: which parts of a plant are effective in what forms, how much you need to take and how often. Many herbs must be taken regularly over an extended period of time

to have a noticeable effect, while others have decreasing effects if taken continuously. I suggest focusing on one plant at a time and gathering as much information about it as you can from various sources. (See "Further Reading" for some of my favorite books on herbs.) Find out through experience what works best for you with your own unique body makeup and inner world.

Following are some suggestions of herbs proven to help with a number of common emotional/mental conditions. These herbs can be used in various ways; the next chapter describes how to make

How to use herbs safely

The majority of herbal remedies are safe and easy to use, and we can use herbs throughout our entire lives. But plants can have a powerful effect on us, so it is important to be aware of the dangers they might pose. While many herbs have been scientifically validated for their positive health benefits, some can also have negative side effects we need to be mindful of. Toxicity can be related to dosage—how much of the plant you are consuming and what your body weight is. It is critical if you are on medications to make sure there are no interactions between these and any herbs you might want to take. For example, California poppy may be contraindicated during pregnancy or with pharmaceuticals. Do your homework and speak to a health care professional.

some basic herbal preparations. Some herbs are easy to grow in your sacred space, and others can be obtained in apothecaries or from reputable suppliers. The table at the end of the chapter summarizes these herbs and their uses, and also mentions a few others you may find helpful. Consider this list just a starting point for your own explorations into the full range of help available from these plant allies.

SOOTHING STRESS

In this day and age, we are plagued by stress. Our body's automatic physiological and psychological response to danger can be a lifesaver when the threat is real, but when this response is provoked by the conditions of daily living, it can create health issues. Working harder than ever, 77 percent of Americans report that stress creates psychological problems in their lives. According to the American Institute of Stress, stress causes 60 percent of human illnesses. Stress can increase the risk of heart disease and heart attack, stroke, and insomnia.

Plant allies that increase the body's ability to resist and restore balance in the face of all kinds of stressors—environmental, physical, emotional, and biological—are called adaptogens. We can use these adaptogens for mental stress, environmental conditions like abrupt temperature changes, and healing from physical trauma: **ashwagandha**, **eleuthero**, **ginseng**, **maitake**, **rhodiola**, and **tulsi**.

EASING ANXIETY

Roughly 40 million adults in the United States have anxiety disorders, and children are becoming more and more affected. I was diagnosed with an anxiety disorder as a young adult, and it has taken me years to understand the whys and how to not be affected. Anxiety leads to a number of mental and physical struggles and is rooted in fear. As a natural response to fear, anxiety can help us, but instead it more often hinders us with

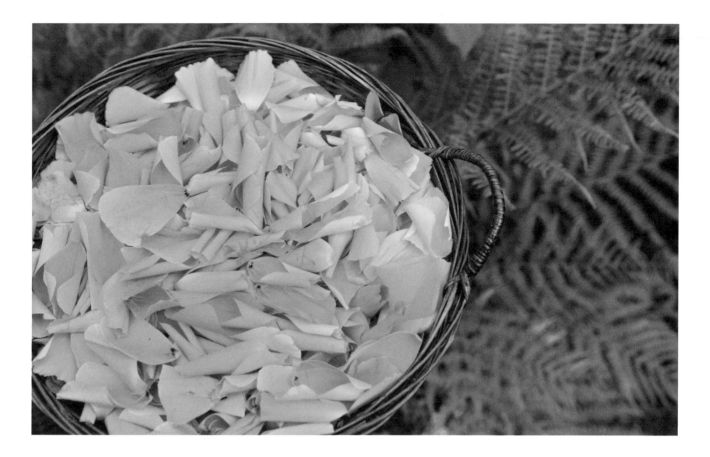

California poppy, considered a weed by many, is a useful herb for easing anxiety and helping us sleep better.

irrational fears of nonexistent problems. We often worry about the future, which is unknown, and we carry memories of negative past experiences into the present unnecessarily.

If you notice anxiety creeping into your life, try getting to know these plant allies, which can help calm fears and anxieties: **ashwagandha**, **California poppy**, **chamomile**, **ginkgo**, **gotu kola**, **hawthorn**, **hops**, **lavender**, **lemon balm**, **linden**, **passionflower**, **rhodiola**, **skullcap**, **tulsi**, and **valerian**.

INVITING RESTFUL SLEEP

Sleep is a necessary pause for our emotions to settle and our bodies to regenerate tissues and organs, but many of us are not getting the seven to eight hours of nightly sleep recommended by the National Institutes of Health. Insomnia and sleep disorders affect tens of millions of adults in the United States and can lead to increased risk of heart disease, obesity, high blood pressure, and diabetes, as well as weakening the immune system and reducing life expectancy.

Herbs are a potent source of help in this realm. For centuries, these plant allies have been known to aid us in achieving sleep and sleeping better, and in guiding our dreams: **ashwagandha**, **bee balm**, **California poppy**, **chamomile**, **ginseng**, **gotu kola**, **hawthorn**, **hops**, **lavender**, **passionflower**, and **valerian**.

CALMING ANGER

Anger is a natural emotion that can stem from being hurt, frustrated, or disappointed. The problem comes when it turns into rage and is directed at others, which can turn into violence, abuse, and trauma. My go-to anger management technique is gardening. There is nothing like shoveling or raking or weeding when you are mad. The earth doesn't mind that extra energy! Any physical activity can help process and release anger, which can actually be a useful and productive energy.

Plants can help with anger as well. The Muskogee tribe used bee balm in a tea or simply crushed for its fragrance when there was lingering or mounting anger in a household. These other plant allies are also known to help calm, stabilize, and soothe us: **burdock**, **chamomile**, **dandelion root**, **lavender**, **linden**, **oat**, **passionflower**, and **skullcap**.

BOOSTING YOUR MOOD

Everyone has a blue mood now and then, and herbs can help lift the cloud. Beyond that, depression is a chronic condition characterized by persistent feelings of sadness, emptiness, fatigue, low energy, and difficulty thinking or sleeping. It makes people more prone to illness such as colds and flus and can have a significant impact on quality of life. Depression affects more than 350 million people globally and is more likely in women (twice as likely as in men), with the average age at onset of thirty-two. One in eight adolescent children have depression. There are differing theories about what causes depression, and there are varying grades of depression.

Dealing with depression is a journey that may require professional help, but these plant allies can help you on that journey: **ashwagandha**, **California poppy**, **chamomile**, **hawthorn**, **lavender**, **lemon balm**, **rhodiola**, **skullcap**, and **St. John's wort**.

COMFORTING HEARTBREAK AND GRIEF

We all live through heartbreak at some point in our lives. The end of a relationship with someone we love, whether through a breakup or death, can be one of the most difficult experiences to endure. Our souls and lives have woven together, and the loss can feel like a tear straight across the heart. As we work on repairing that emotional tear, it can be a struggle to get through the physical pain, the

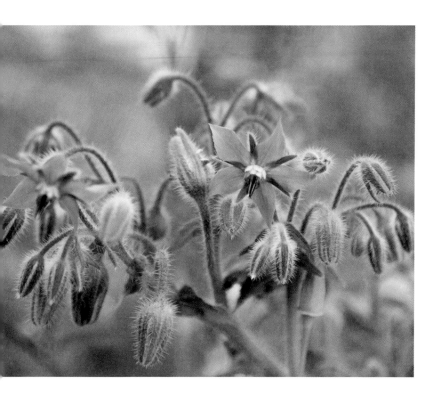

Borage is known to relax the nervous system and help with grief.

and affect us dramatically, especially if it is not addressed. Post-traumatic stress disorder (PTSD) affects 20 million people in the United States. According to the National Center for PTSD, a greater percentage of women than men are likely to be affected; rape is the biggest trigger, and childhood abuse leads to a strong likelihood of developing PTSD later in life.

Trauma can take work with a professional to overcome. These plant allies can help by soothing the nervous system and alleviating anxiety, stress, insomnia, digestive issues, and anger: **chamomile, ginseng, gotu kola, lavender, St. John's wort, and valerian.**

emotional longing, the confusion, and the rollercoaster of feelings.

For thousands of years, people have turned to these plant allies for help: **borage, burdock, California poppy, chamomile, eleuthero, hawthorn, lavender, lemon balm, St. John's wort, tulsi,** and **violet.**

ALLEVIATING TRAUMA

Different from stress, trauma is the result of an experience or event that is often life threatening. It can also come from physical, psychological, or sexual abuse, which causes the nervous system to go into fight-or-flight mode. This is a normal response, but it can be stored in the body

KEEPING YOUR BRAIN HEALTHY

Several herbs can help support our cognitive functions—our ability to focus, have mental clarity, and retain our memory. A cognitive tea formulation can be great for students who are studying hard, for those working under a deadline, and as we age and lose memory or concentration. These plant allies can help: **ashwagandha, eleuthero, ginkgo, ginseng, gotu kola, oat, rhodiola,** and **tulsi.**

Plant allies for common emotional/mental conditions

Common name, *botanical name*	Benefits	How to use
ashwagandha, *Withania somnifera*	Adaptogen; balances body systems, increases energy and concentration, reduces anxiety and stress.	Use the dried root in infusions, decoctions, and tinctures, or in capsule form.
bee balm, *Monarda didyma**	Quells anger and promotes restful sleep.	Use the dried leaf, stem, and flowers in teas and tinctures; add fresh flowers to salads.
borage, *Borago officinalis**	Relaxes the nervous system; helps stress, exhaustion, and grief.	Use fresh flowers and leaves in teas, tinctures, and oils; add fresh flowers to salads and fresh leaves to soups.
burdock, *Arctium lappa***	Balances the system, promotes strength and vitality, helps maintain a stable internal environment.	Use the dried root in decoctions and tinctures, or in capsule form.
California poppy, *Eschscholzia californica**	Relieves anxiety, promotes healthy sleep, relaxes muscle spasms.	Use the fresh root or whole plant in teas and tinctures; add fresh flowers to salads and desserts.
chamomile, *Matricaria recutita**	Calms anxiety, soothes anger and nervousness, promotes relaxation.	Use the dried flowering tops in teas and tinctures.
dandelion, *Taraxacum officinale***	Cleanses the liver and calms anger.	Use fresh leaves and roots in teas and tinctures; add fresh leaves to salads and soups.
eleuthero, *Eleutherococcus senticosus*	Adaptogen; improves mental alertness and memory, reduces fatigue, increases stamina and resilience.	Use the dried root in teas and tinctures or in capsule form.
ginkgo, *Ginkgo biloba**	Improves circulation, protects memory, increases calmness.	Use the dried leaves in teas and tinctures, or in capsule form.
ginseng, *Panax ginseng*	Adaptogen; promotes resistance to stress and fatigue, enhances cognition and mood, improves sleep quality.	Use the dried root in infusions or in capsule form.
gotu kola, *Centella asiatica*	Aids mental clarity, promotes restful sleep, reduces anxiety and nervousness.	Use fresh or dried leaves in teas and tinctures; add fresh leaves to salads and other dishes; juice along with other vegetables.

hawthorn, *Crataegus* spp.*	Opens and mends the heart, calms the nervous system, reduces anxiety, helps with insomnia.	Use the ripe berries in jams, jellies, and syrups; use the dried leaves, flowers, and berries in teas and tinctures or in capsule form.
hops, *Humulus lupulus**	Soothes anxiety and excitability, promotes sleep and relaxation.	Use fresh or dried flowers in teas and tinctures or in capsule form; use dried flowers in dream pillows and bathwater.
lavender, *Lavandula angustifolia**	Lifts the spirits, relaxes the body, promotes restful sleep, helps soothe anxiety.	Use dried flower spikes and leaves in teas, tinctures, and infused or essential oils; add dried flowers to dream pillows, potpourris, and desserts; add oil to bathwater.
lemon balm, *Melissa officinalis**	Calms the nerves, lifts the spirits, comforts the heart.	Use the fresh leaves in teas, tinctures, and infused water; add fresh leaves to salads, butters, cooked dishes, sauces, and marinades.
linden, *Tilia* spp.*	Calms the nerves, soothes mental stress and anxiety.	Use dried flowers in teas and tinctures, or in capsule form; add fresh flowers to bathwater.
maitake, *Grifola frondosa*	Adaptogen; helps in reducing stress and boosting immune function.	Use dried fungus in tincture or capsule form.
oat, *Avena sativa**	Relaxes the nervous system, promotes a sense of calm, boosts attention and concentration.	Use the dried stems, leaves, and grains in teas and tinctures, and in capsule form.
passionflower, *Passiflora incarnata**	Relieves anxiety and helps with insomnia.	Use the dried flowers, leaves, and stems in teas and tinctures, or in capsule form.
rhodiola, *Rhodiola rosea*	Adaptogen; promotes mental clarity, counteracts stress and fatigue, calms anxiety.	Use the root fresh or dried in teas and tinctures, or take the powdered root in capsule form.
skullcap, *Scutellaria lateriflora**	Soothes the nervous system, calms a restless mind, improves mood.	Use dried leaves and stems in teas and tinctures.
St. John's wort, *Hypericum perforatum**	Soothes the nervous system and helps with mild to moderate depression.	Use the dried flowers in teas, tinctures, and infused oils.
tulsi, *Ocimum tenuiflorum**	Adaptogen; counteracts the effects of stress, eases anxiety, improves mental clarity and memory.	Use the dried leaves and flowers in teas and tinctures, and in capsule form; add fresh leaves to cooked dishes.
valerian, *Valeriana officinalis**	Calms the nervous system and promotes healthy sleep.	Use the root fresh in a tincture, or take the powdered root in capsule form.
violet, *Viola odorata**	Calms the heart and soothes the spirit.	Use fresh or dried leaves in teas and tinctures; add the flowers to a salad or use to garnish a soup or dessert.

*Described in greater detail in the previous chapter.
**Described in greater detail under "The Wisdom of Weeds" earlier in this chapter.

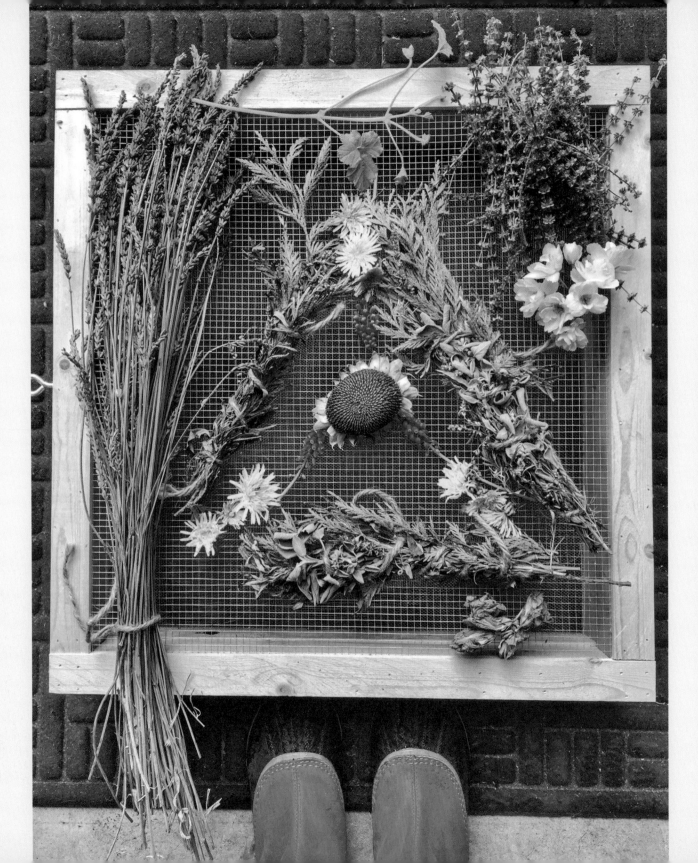

Growing Your Own Apothecary

Herbs harvested from a sanctuary garden form the basis of a home apothecary.

RIGHT I incorporate herbs everywhere I have space, and I know the plants will thrive because I give them the conditions they do best in.

It is always best to grow your own beneficial plants if and when possible to get the maximum health benefits. Growing your own plants in your sanctuary garden ensures that no chemicals were used and the plants are in their freshest state when you harvest them. Fresh is best, but we don't always have access to the freshest harvest year-round, so creating an apothecary is a great way to save plants—and money. You can prepare your own remedies with just a few supplies and with fresh herbs or dried.

Your Herb Garden

Many culinary and medicinal herb plants are available at specialty nurseries or through catalogs. Most herbs prefer a sunny spot and can be located next to or near annual vegetable gardens. Some herbs can be grown inside on a sunny windowsill or on a deck in containers.

Be sure to give them enough space from other plants along with the soil conditions and sun exposure they prefer. If you use a large quantity of a plant, consider working it into your garden in several spots.

Gardens designed specifically for herbs can be any shape and size, depending on your own preferences. You can create a medicinal herb garden around a specific theme. For instance, a tea garden

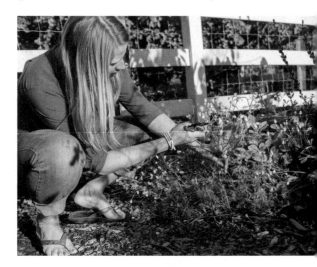

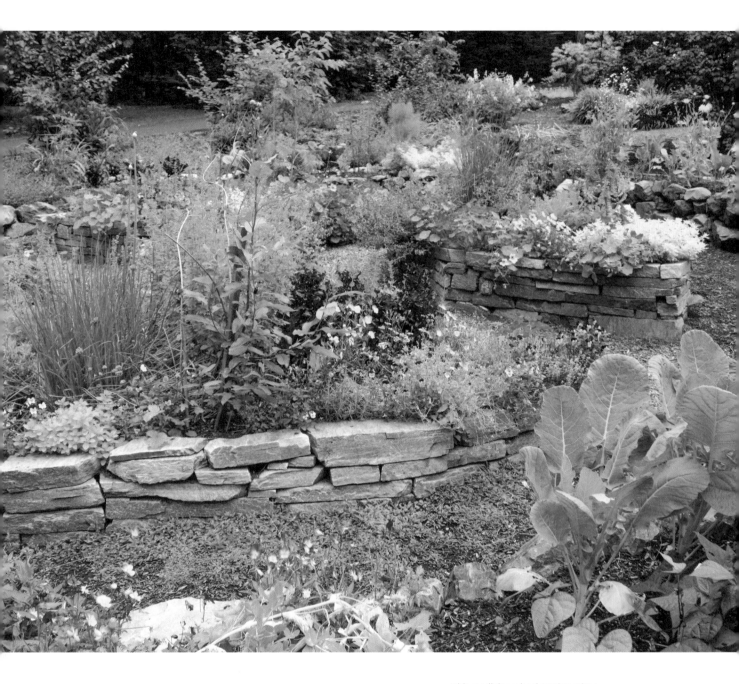

This medicine wheel garden mixes
medicinal herbs with edibles.

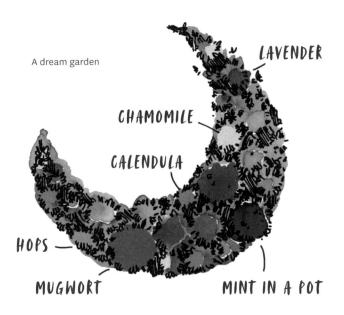

A dream garden

LAVENDER

CHAMOMILE

CALENDULA

HOPS

MUGWORT

MINT IN A POT

containing plants to treat what ails you is a great place to start. A dream garden can contain herbs known to promote healthy sleep and nourishing dreams. What shape do you want it to take? How about the shape of a crescent moon?

Mushroom Gardens

I recommend growing some mushrooms in your sacred space for their ecological and medicinal value. Many mushrooms are edible, and more and more scientific research is discovering how medically and

How to save seeds for propagation

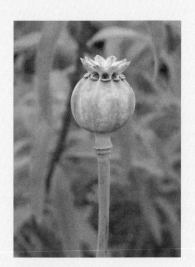

Poppy seed heads contain thousands of small seeds that are easy to collect and disperse.

Collecting seeds to start the next generation of plants in your sacred space is a great way to save money, feel empowered, and stay closely connected to the plants you are growing and will be using. Some easy herbs to start with are borage, calendula, California poppy, and echinacea.

Notice the plants that are healthy and disease free, and pick their seed-pods when they have dried and are beginning to open. For plants with fragile seedpods, you can put a paper bag over the seedpods and secure it with a twist tie before harvesting so that you capture all of the seed. Split the seedpods and shake all the seeds out into a basin or bowl, then spread them out on clean paper in a warm, dry place for about a week. Pack them in airtight labeled jars or bags and store in a cool, dry place.

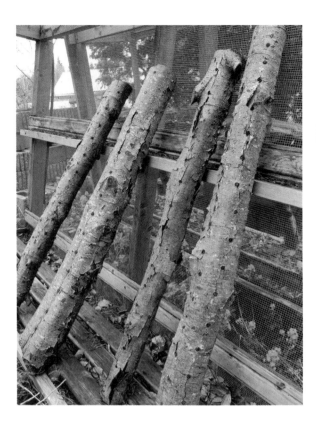

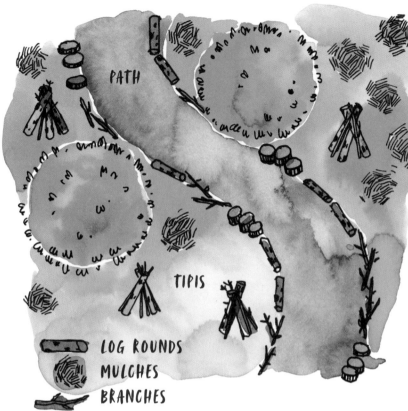

PATH

TIPIS

LOG ROUNDS
MULCHES
BRANCHES

Placing plugs of fungus in branches drilled with holes is an easy way to grow a variety of edible and medicinal mushrooms.

ABOVE RIGHT A mushroom garden

ecologically beneficial some can actually be. Not only can some mushrooms restore the damaged earth by absorbing toxins and cleansing water, but some also have antiviral, antibacterial, and cancer-fighting properties. Mycologist Paul Stamets writes, "Mushrooms are miniature pharmaceutical factories, and of the thousands of mushroom species in nature, our ancestors and modern scientists have identified several dozen that have a unique combination of talents that improve our health."

Several edible mushrooms are easy to grow using materials found at home and spores in sawdust or in plugs ordered from fungi suppliers such as Mushroom

Mountain (mushroommountain.com) and Fungi Perfecti (fungi.com). Shady spaces are the best places to grow mushrooms. Log rounds and long branches used to line forest paths provide great habitat for plugs to spawn. A tipi made of branches can grow different types of fungus and makes a great focal point. Woodchip mulches and other biomass (such as leaves and straw) can host different kinds of mushrooms, depending on the parent material.

Some mushrooms are poisonous, so it is important to gather information as you decide what to grow and use, just as you would for any other plant. Before you

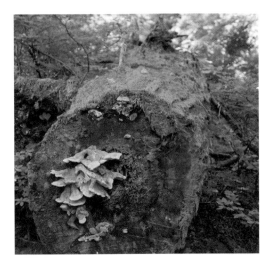

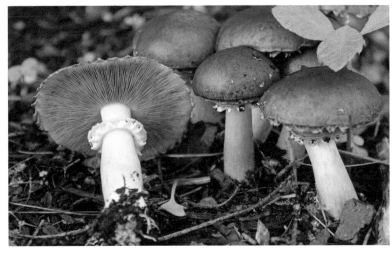

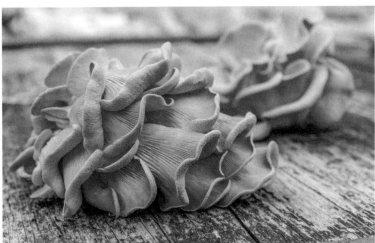

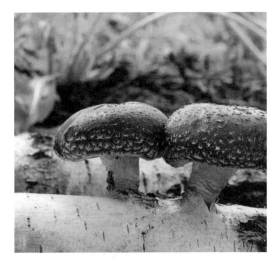

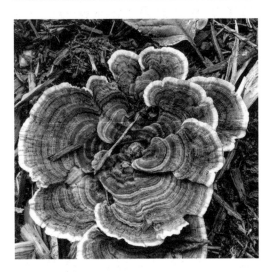

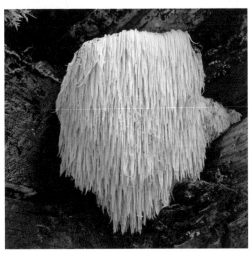

CLOCKWISE FROM TOP LEFT

Chicken of the woods, *Laetiporus* species

Wine caps, *Stropharia rugosoannulata*

Shiitake, *Lentinula edodes*

Lion's mane, *Hericium erinaceus*

Turkey tail, *Trametes versicolor*

Oyster mushrooms, *Pleurotus* species

Easy-to-grow mushrooms

Common name	Botanical name	Type	Growing medium
chicken of the woods	*Laetiporus* spp.	edible	hardwoods such as oak
lion's mane	*Hericium erinaceus*	edible and medicinal	hardwoods such as elm, maple, oak, poplar
oyster	*Pleurotus* spp.	edible	hardwoods such as poplar
shiitake	*Lentinula edodes*	edible	hardwoods such as alder, maple, oak
turkey tail	*Trametes versicolor*	medicinal	Douglas-fir, and hardwoods such as alder, aspen, beech, birch, cherry, locust, oak, plum, poplar, and walnut
wine caps	*Stropharia rugosoannulata*	edible	hardwoods

consume any mushroom, make positively sure you have identified it accurately. You can find a list of local mycological societies, which may be able to help you, on the North American Mycological Association website at namyo.org.

Wildcrafting and Ethical Harvesting

Some herbs such as nettle and lamb's quarters are easy to find growing alongside roads and in uncultivated areas. As harvesting wild plants like these for human use—a practice known as wildcrafting—has risen in popularity, the risk to plant populations of taking too much has also grown. A basic rule of thumb is to never take more than a third of the harvestable parts from a plant; leave a third for other fauna and a third for the plant itself.

Here are some other points of etiquette:

* Never harvest plants from a property when you don't know who owns it. Trespassing is a crime. Most people don't mind if you want to harvest plants from their site, but just make sure to ask first. Even on public land

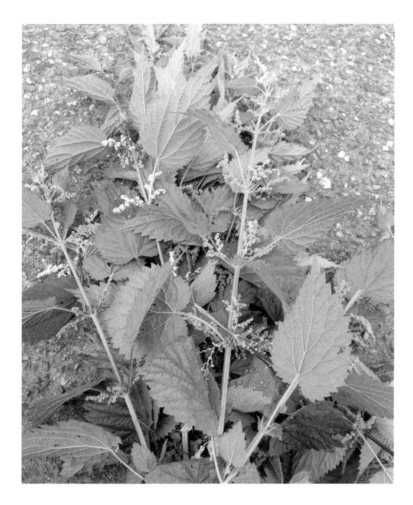

I took less than a third of this nettle found growing wild near my home.

cultures, objects or elements such as pennies or cornmeal are given to the plant in appreciation.

✳ Beware of toxins. This is especially true of plants growing alongside roads and in ditches, where residue from pesticides, car exhaust, and stormwater runoff can be present. If a plant has been exposed to or sprayed with herbicides, the leaves will usually look discolored and wilted. However, many pesticides are persistent in the soil for several years, so the more you know about a site's history, the better.

Basics of Processing Plants

Processing plants for your apothecary starts with harvesting healthy and clean plant material. Depending on the plant and the medicine you want to make, you may be gathering leaves, flowers, roots, or bark. As a rule of thumb, the best time to harvest is in the morning after the dew dries and before the heat of the day. Clean this material as necessary to dislodge soil, insects, and dead or diseased leaves. If you are purchasing plant material, be sure to ask your supplier where the plants were harvested and if any chemicals were used in growing them. Nasty products such as fumigants, heavy metal fertilizers,

there are rules and regulations that must be followed.

✳ Ask the plant for permission as well. Consider its vigor and health, and whether there are more like it nearby. If it is struggling and the population is small, it may not reproduce easily or thrive if you take from it.

✳ Share your gratitude. Say thank you and make an offering. In many

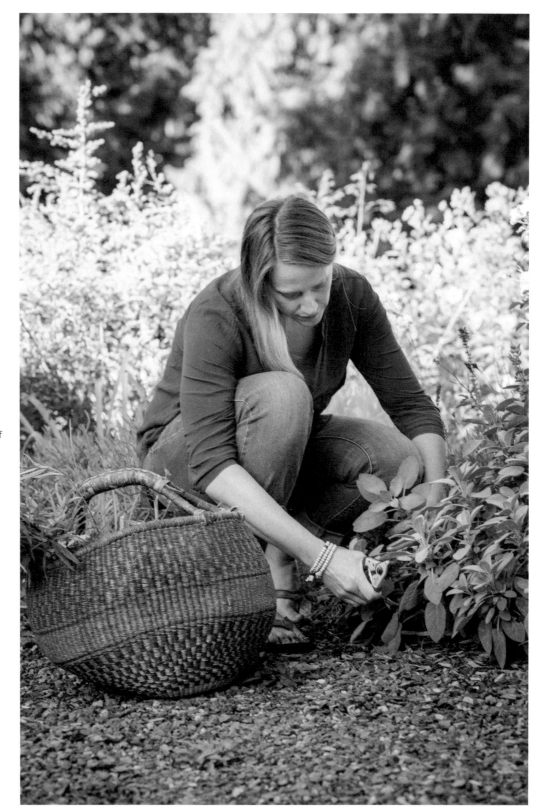

Harvesting plants is best done when the potency of the plant's constituents is the highest, generally in the morning after the dew dries and before the heat of the day.

Make space for drying, processing, and storage

When I first started making my own plant medicine, the kitchen and every closet was full of plant material drying, hanging from the ceiling. Open any cupboard and you would find stacked jars of herbs and supplies. I was running out of room and constantly had a disorganized mess on my hands. As my passion for plant medicine grew, so did my need for an organized system to bring plants from the garden inside, to dry them, to process them, and to store the herbs and finished products, whether it was tea blends, infused oils, tinctures, or what have you.

This was tricky as I had downsized into a smaller home and had little room to spare. I chose two areas: a spot in my garage for drying and processing, and a repurposed coat closet in the hallway between the front door and the kitchen to store finished products and supplies for easy access. The drying and processing area gets messy, so I needed an area that was easy to clean. For the indoor storage, I could have built or repurposed a piece of furniture, but I liked the idea of having built-in shelves and being able to shut the door.

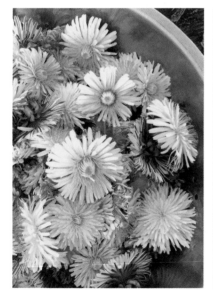

Dandelion flowers have been collected for their petals.

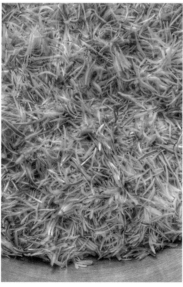

The tedious task of plucking petals can be turned into a therapeutic meditation.

pesticides, herbicides, fungicides, insecticides, and sulfur are all known to be used in the worldwide herbal markets.

Dry your herbs in an area that is free from moisture, has good air circulation, and is out of direct sunlight, preferably dark. Some herbs are best hung to dry, while others dry better spread out on a mesh like a window screen. A food dehydrator can be a good investment for drying herb parts quickly while retaining their valuable properties. I have an 8-foot-long wire strung in my garage to hang herbs on, a multilevel hanging mesh screen, a variety of window screens, and

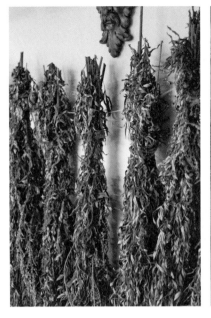

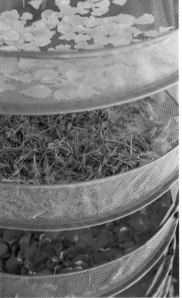

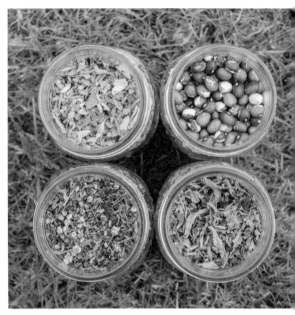

Bundled herbs are hung on a string in a dry area out of direct sunlight.

This multilevel mesh dryer works well for drying loose plant materials like leaves and petals.

Dried plant materials are stored in mason jars.

a solar dehydrator. Depending on the plant, humidity, and air temperature, it may take anywhere from a few days to several weeks for herbs to dry thoroughly. Make sure air can flow through the plant material and check it often, moving and rotating the material if needed.

Once the plants have dried, one of my favorite chores is to strip the leaves off the stems so that they can easily be stored and used. Often I will start by placing the plant material in a large paper bag or a sieve to break it apart. I wear a dust mask, or at least a bandana to cover my mouth, as it can be a dusty experience.

You can use a variety of storage containers to keep your herbs as fresh as possible. The container needs to be airtight and easy to label. I started with a mix-and-match apothecary, saving jars and containers from everything I had on hand. I prefer mason jars for the ease of

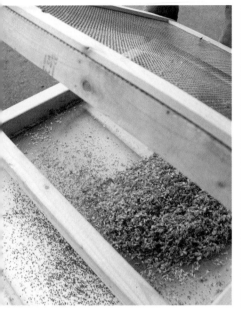

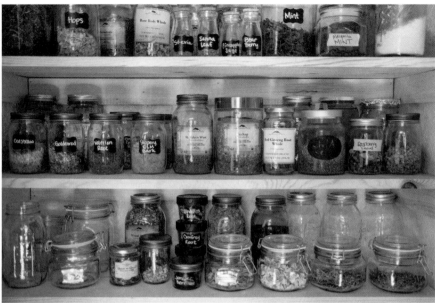

Screens with different sizes of mesh are great for processing plants into smaller pieces or to separate seeds out.

Be sure to label all the containers holding dried plant material ready for use.

cleaning, reuse, and storage for dried or liquid material. You can use plastics and paper also, which may be cheaper but may also not be ideal for some herbs. Be sure to label each container with the plant name and date of harvest. Expect fresh herbs that have been processed correctly to last about a year; they will lose their color, and their potency will decrease with time.

Introduction to Making Medicines

Making herbal medicines is no more complicated than following a recipe in your kitchen. Although you can buy teas, tinctures, salves, ointments, and essential oils at the store, making them yourself can be an enjoyable and empowering part of the healing process. Supplies you'll want to have on hand include pots and pans

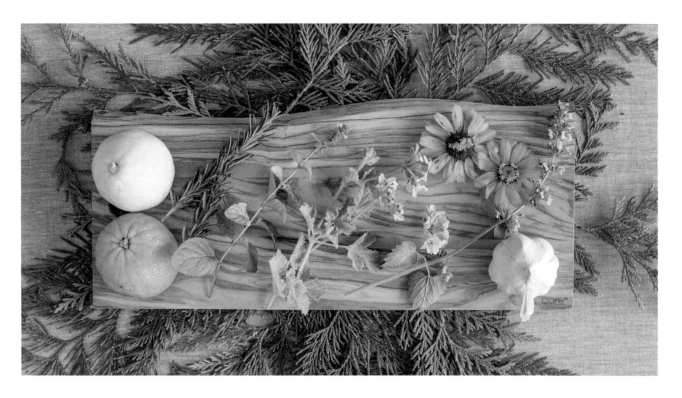

You can use a variety of plants to make teas, tinctures, sprays, oils, salves, and creams.

(uncoated stainless steel is best), Pyrex measuring cups, a small kitchen scale, a food processor or blender, strainers and infusers like tea balls, airtight containers, labels, and funnels.

You'll use herbs to make these kinds of remedies:

* infusions—teas made the most common way, by pouring boiling water over fresh or dried leaves or flowers and then straining out the herbs

* decoctions—teas made by boiling down and concentrating the hard or woody parts of an herb, like the bark, roots, and seeds, and then straining them out

* tinctures—solutions made by grinding and soaking fresh or dried herbs in an alcohol or vinegar solvent and then straining out the herbs

* oils—oils slowly infused with dried herbs that can be used externally or incorporated into salves and creams

* salves and creams—compounds of infused oils with water and wax as a moisturizing base to apply externally to skin

* compresses—pads or cloths saturated with herbal teas that can be applied hot or cold to wounds, burns, infections, sprains, and muscle aches

Following are step-by-step instructions for each kind of remedy.

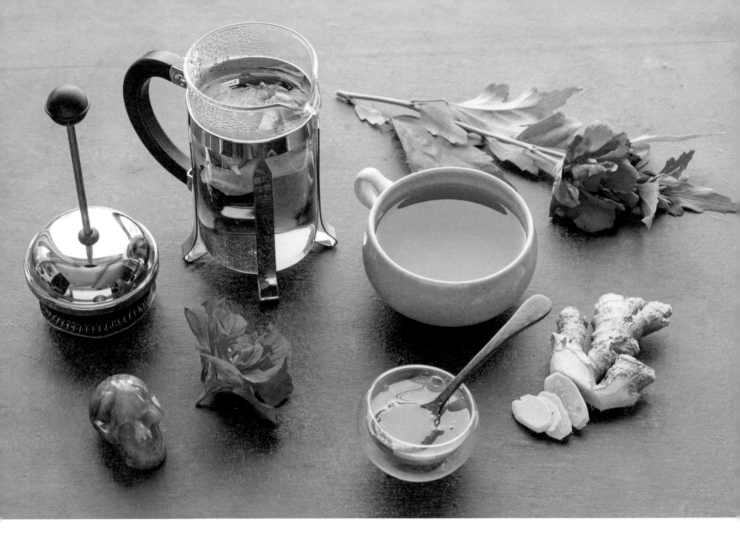

Herbal teas are easy to make and blend with your favorite ingredients.

TEAS, FRESH AND DRIED

Teas use boiling water to extract the valuable compounds from an herb, concentrating them in a form that is easy to drink hot or cold. To make an infusion, you can generally pour 10 liquid ounces of boiling water over 2 to 3 ounces of fresh herb or 1 ounce of dried herb, and more or less for a stronger or weaker tea. Use purified water and let the herbs (flowers, leaves, and small stems) steep for ten or twenty minutes before pouring the liquid through a fine-mesh strainer to remove the plant parts. For a decoction, use the same proportions but place the plant parts (bark, roots, and seeds) and water in a saucepan and bring to a boil. Reduce the temperature and simmer the herbs for twenty minutes to an hour before straining out the plant parts and drinking the tea.

145

GROWING YOUR OWN APOTHECARY

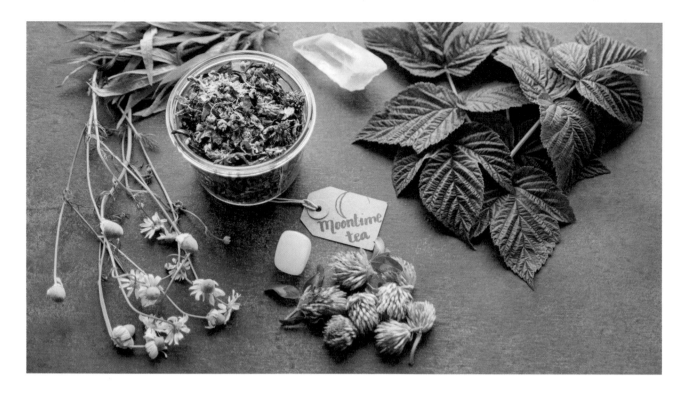

Moontime tea is my favorite tea for relaxation and helps ease the symptoms associated with women's monthly cycle, including cramps, bloating, and mood swings.

Mood Lifter Tea

2–3 tablespoons fresh or 1 tablespoon dried lemon balm leaf

2–3 teaspoons fresh or 1 teaspoon dried tulsi

2–3 teaspoons fresh or 1 teaspoon dried hibiscus

4 cups purified water

Place the herbs in an infuser or container. Bring the water to a boil and pour over the herbs. Let the mixture steep, covered, for ten to twenty minutes. Strain into a cup and drink up to 5 cups a day.

Moontime Tea

4–5 tablespoons fresh or 2 tablespoons dried raspberry leaf

2–3 teaspoons fresh or 1 teaspoon dried mugwort

2–3 teaspoons fresh or 1 teaspoon dried chamomile

2–3 teaspoons fresh or 1 teaspoon dried red clover

2–3 teaspoons fresh or 1 teaspoon dried skullcap

4 cups purified water

Place the herbs in an infuser or container. Bring the water to a boil and pour over the herbs. Let the mixture steep, covered, for ten to twenty minutes. Strain into a cup and drink up to 5 cups a day.

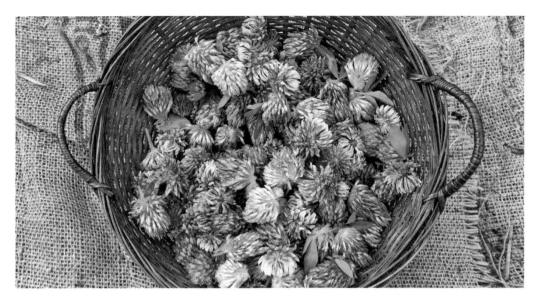

Red clover is a common "weed" packed with potent medicinal constituents and can be used in teas and tinctures.

TINCTURES

The medicinal constituents of herbs dissolve very well in alcohol, which is the base used to make tinctures. Tinctures stored away from heat and light can preserve the medicinal properties of herbs for a year or more, and they are easy to take directly by mouth with a dropper or stirred into water. The basic method of preparation is to grind or chop up fresh or dried herbs, add them to a solution of alcohol, let the mixture sit for two to three weeks in a cool and dark place, and strain out the herbs. Vodka and ethyl alcohol are the two preferred forms of alcohol to use when making tinctures.

Red Clover Tincture

Red clover is known as a general wellness herb and blood purifier. It may help with menopausal symptoms but has estrogen-like effects so should not be taken by women with a history of breast cancer.

2 to 3 ounces fresh or 1 ounce dried red clover flowers, finely chopped

5 liquid ounces 160-proof vodka (if using fresh flowers) or 100-proof vodka (if using dried)

In a clean glass jar, combine the flowers and vodka. Add more vodka if necessary until the flowers are completely covered by the vodka and then some. Tighten the lid and shake lightly. Store in a dark place for four to six weeks, shaking daily. Strain the liquid into a small amber dropper bottle, squeezing the flowers to get the last drops out. Take 40 to 60 drops in water three times a day.

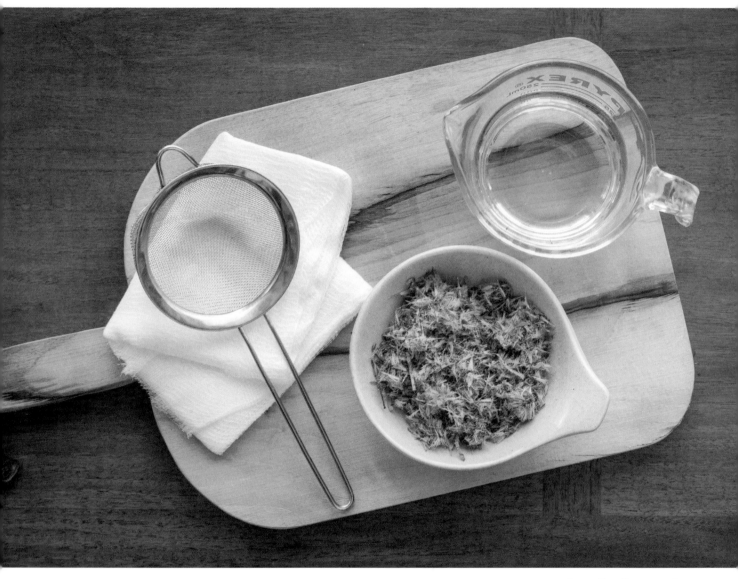

For making oils, you need plant material, oil, a strainer, cheesecloth, and a glass jar (not pictured).

OILS

Herbs can be infused into oils, and these herbal oils can be taken internally or used externally for body care. They can also be used in making salves and creams. Cold-pressed, unrefined organic oils without additives are ideal. Coconut oil is the best multipurpose oil, but it does solidify at 76 degrees F. Olive, sunflower, grapeseed, and avocado oil are readily available and versatile. Almond and jojoba are also good choices.

The basic procedure is to combine a handful of finely ground herbs (leaves, flowers, roots, bark, and/or seeds) with a similar amount of oil in a clean glass jar with the herbs completely submerged in the oil. (Dried herbs are preferred here as fresh herbs will sometimes ferment, depending on the herb.) Then you store the tightly lidded jar for two to four weeks, shaking the jar daily. Heat speeds up the process, so put the jar on a sunny windowsill if you can. Filter the oil through cheesecloth or muslin into an amber bottle and label it with the contents and date before storing it in a dark place.

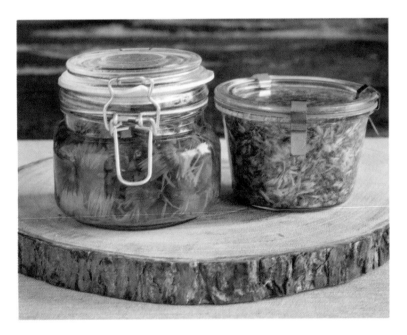

Arnica (right) and calendula (left) have been infused into these oils.

Calendula-Infused Oil

Calendula-infused oil is easy to make and can be applied directly to soothe rashes, sunburns, and skin irritations, or it can be used later in a salve or cream.

wilted fresh calendula flowers
equal amount of a cold-pressed,
  unrefined organic oil

Harvest the flowers at midday and let them sit for twenty-four to forty-eight hours so there is no longer moisture on the petals. Then strip off the petals and fill a clean glass jar with them. Add enough oil to cover them completely. Stir it and seal it. Let it sit on a sunny windowsill for two to four weeks, gently shaking it every day. Then use cheesecloth to strain the oil into another jar for storage in a dark place. Wring out the cheesecloth to squeeze out as much oil as possible.

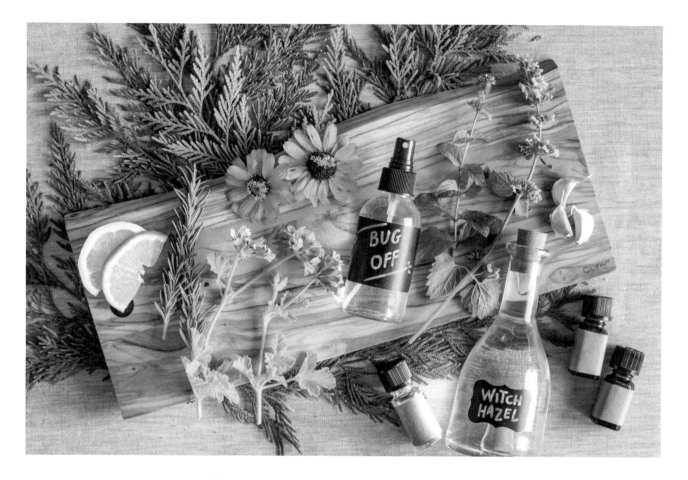

Bug-Off Spray

To ward off unwanted insects in your home, on your pets, or on you, try this simple recipe. When selecting the plant to use, consider testing first for fragrance and potential skin irritation.

4 ounces water

4 ounces witch hazel

50–60 drops oil infused with one of these plants: basil, catnip, cedar, chamomile, chives, eucalyptus, feverfew, garlic, geraniums, lemon, lemon balm, marigolds, rosemary, sage, or spearmint

Fill an 8-ounce spray bottle halfway with water, then top it off with witch hazel. Add the drops of infused oil and shake well.

Aromatherapy and essential oils

Essential oils are extracted from herbs to highly concentrate the compounds that give the herbs their characteristic scent. It takes a lot of an herb to make a little of an essential oil, so they are expensive and should be used ethically. A little essential oil goes a long way: a few drops can be diluted in water to spritz a room, dropped into bath water to make it fragrant, or placed in boiling water or a steamer to diffuse into a room. Essential oils have proven health benefits, including lifting mood and improving sleep, and aromatherapy is used in some hospitals and clinics as a complementary medicine. These oils should not be taken internally without professional medical advice. If you use them on your skin, you should dilute them first with an oil like those used for infused oils.

You can use essential oils to scent infused oils and salves you prepare. You can also give yourself all the benefits of aromatherapy by planting fragrant herbs and then crushing a leaf or two to inhale. Whenever I pass by rosemary and lavender in my garden, I rub my hands over the shrubs and then cup my hands to my face and inhale the living botanical perfumes.

Here are my five favorite aromatherapy plants to grow:

* bee balm—calms the nerves, reduces nausea, reduces cold symptoms

* chamomile—reduces anxiety, promotes sleep, is anti-inflammatory

* lavender—reduces anxiety, promotes relaxation, promotes cell regeneration

* peppermint—energizes, relieves nausea, alleviates migraines, helps concentration

* rosemary—enhances long-term memory, aids alertness, alleviates migraines

SALVES AND CREAMS

Salves, creams, and lotions are an ideal way to deliver the healing benefits of herbs to irritated skin. They make use of your infused oils and add in water and/or beeswax to create a moisturizing base that's more convenient to apply than just the oil itself. Salves are made of oils and wax; they are typically somewhat solid and last longer than creams and lotions. Creams and lotions are mixtures of oil and water, with a little wax added for body. They spoil easily and should be kept refrigerated if not used within more than a few days.

Salves and creams are simple and fun to create, and they make great gifts. As with teas, you can experiment and find a recipe that suits you using plants that can help treat your skin ailments and just keep your skin healthy. I make salves for sun exposure, tattoo healing, and general skin health.

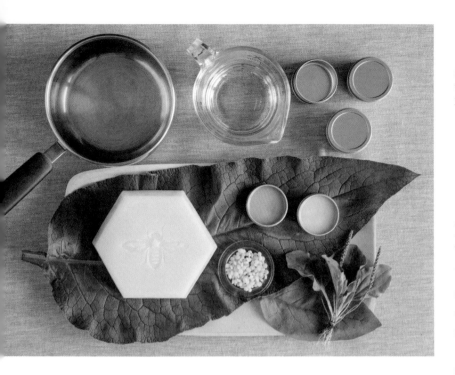

Salves are made with wax and oils infused with your choice of herbs.

Basic Facial Cream

This facial cream can be made with herbs and oils of your choice. Be sure to test any of these ingredients on your face for a reaction before including in a cream.

¾ ounce beeswax
¼ cup almond oil, infused before-
   hand with herbs of your choice
¼ cup coconut oil or cocoa butter
1 cup aloe vera gel
essential oil(s) of your choice
vitamin A or E oils if desired

In a double boiler, melt the beeswax, almond oil, and coconut oil together. Pour them into a blender and let cool to room temperature. In another container, mix the aloe vera gel and essential oil(s). Once the oils in the blender are cool, start to blend slowly and pour in the aloe vera gel mixture. Blend until you like the consistency and color, then pour into clean or sterilized containers. Store in your fridge and use with clean hands.

Healing Salve

2 cups olive or almond oil, infused before-
   hand with herbs of your choice, such as
   plantain leaf, comfrey leaf, or calendula
¼ cup beeswax pastilles or car-
   nauba wax for vegan recipes
essential oil(s) of your choice

In a double boiler, combine the ingredients and bring up the temperature slowly, stirring until the wax melts. To test, dip a spoon into the mixture and put it in the fridge to set. You can add more oil or wax to get the consistency you desire, then pour into a glass jar or tins.

COMPRESSES

A compress is a pad or cloth saturated with an herbal tea and then applied to heal and restore the skin or relieve inflammation or pain in joints and muscles. Hot compresses can be kept warm with a hot water bottle to soothe aches and infections; cold compresses can be kept cold with an ice pack to soothe itching or burning pain. You can use any kind of absorbent material to make a compress, but washcloths are ideal; pieces of old flannel sheets and old T-shirts also work. The basic procedure is to cut or fold the cloth to be slightly larger than the affected area, soak the compress in a strong tea, squeeze the cloth until it is thoroughly wet but not dripping, and apply the compress to the affected area.

Ginger Compress

A ginger compress can relieve muscular aches and pains with its natural anti-inflammatory effect. Apply a ginger compress hot several times a day.

2 ounces fresh or 1 ounce dried ginger root
4 cups purified water
washcloth or other absorbent cloth

In a saucepan, combine the ginger root and water and bring to a boil, then simmer for thirty minutes. Let the tea cool to a tolerable temperature, dip the cloth in, and then squeeze it out until it is wet but not dripping. Apply to the painful area and cover with a small plastic bag or plastic wrap and a small towel. Leave in place for twenty to thirty minutes.

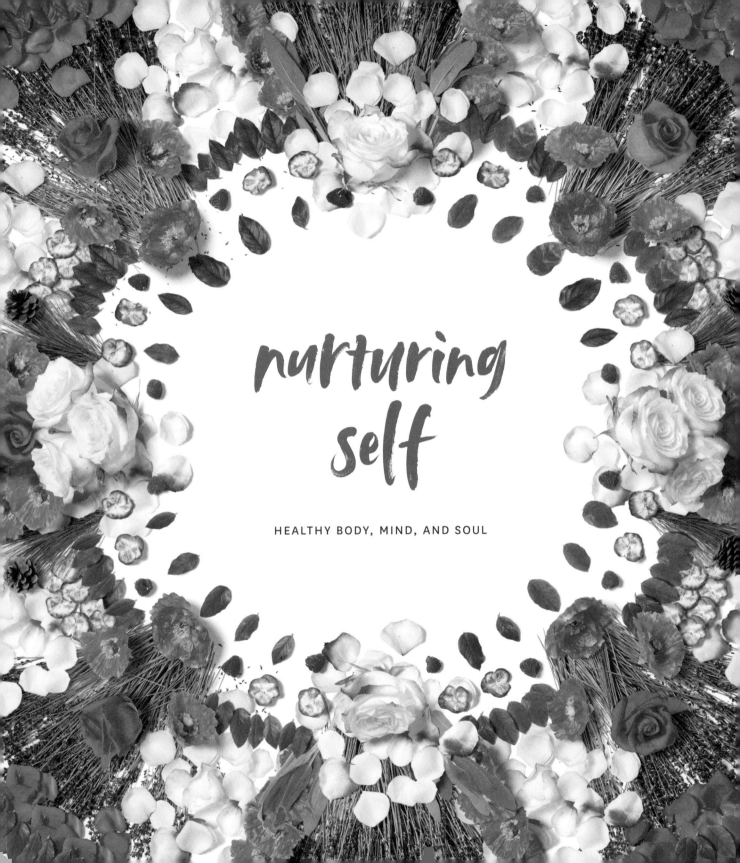

nurturing self

HEALTHY BODY, MIND, AND SOUL

"Wonderful how completely everything in wild nature fits into us, as if truly part and parent of us. The sun shines not on us but in us. The rivers flow not past, but through us, thrilling, tingling, vibrating every fiber and cell of the substance of our bodies, making them glide and sing. The trees wave and the flowers bloom in our bodies as well as our souls, and every bird song, wind song, and tremendous storm song of the rocks in the heart of the mountains is our song, our very own, and sings our love."

JOHN MUIR, "MOUNTAIN THOUGHTS"

Our ancestors were intrinsically wild and natural. Nowadays it seems like we're so far removed from nature, it's easy to forget that we are still interconnected with all living things. To rewild ourselves means to return back to a life where we have nurturing relationships with the natural world—the earth, plants, animals, and self, much like it was long before the industrialized and technological culture we live in today. We can still enjoy the benefits of domestication, but moving back toward our wildness gives us more resilience and skills to thrive, naturally. Our bodies and our minds have been polluted

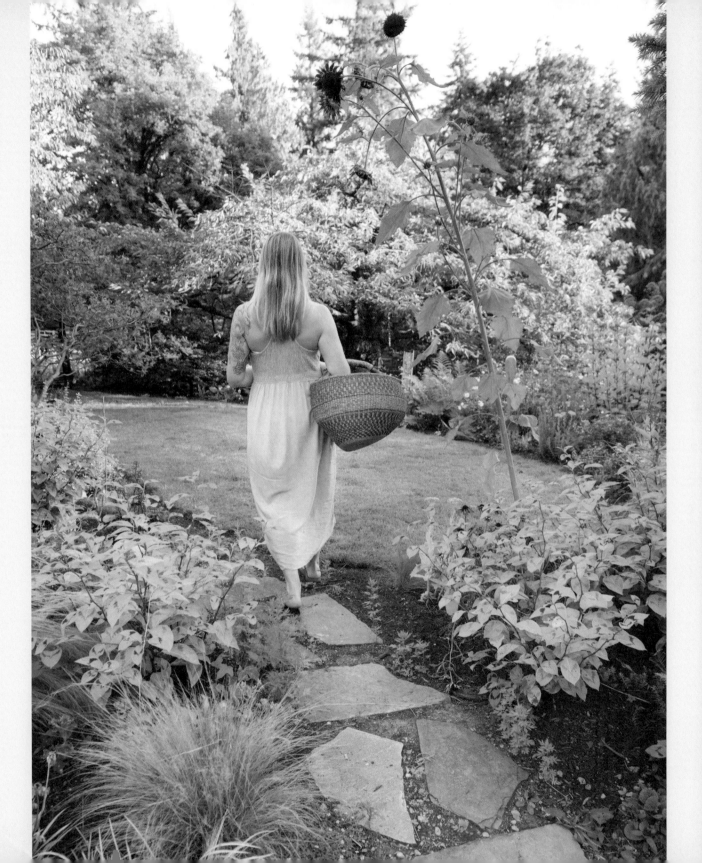

with modern toxins, and it's time to detox. To live simply and with a healthy lifestyle means returning to who we are at the core. We are, in fact, nature.

Nature will nurture us if we, in turn, nurture nature. That includes nurturing our selves. Although we are surrounded with consumer products and technology, we are wired just like other mammals, and our basic needs are very simple: eating healthy food, keeping our bodies strong through exercise, getting enough sleep, staying mentally sharp and focused, being emotionally intelligent in connecting to other humans, and maintaining a caring relationship with the natural world. Being devoted to health can be challenging if it hasn't been a priority in your life, as old habits die hard. It often takes something like an illness or trauma for people to make changes, but you can try to avoid that and consciously choose to take care of yourself.

Time spent in our garden sanctuary can help us rewild ourselves and bring wellness to body, mind, and soul.

You will find suggestions here to help you care for yourself by incorporating simple, nature-based routines every day. Ideally, you will discover your own best practices for benefiting from the sacred space you have created and the plant allies you have cultivated. You will come to rely on your sanctuary for developing emotional and physical resiliency, feeling safe, and finding clarity and strength. Your soul, your heart, your nervous system, your entire self can relax. Feeling connected to yourself and committed to your own well-being is the first step.

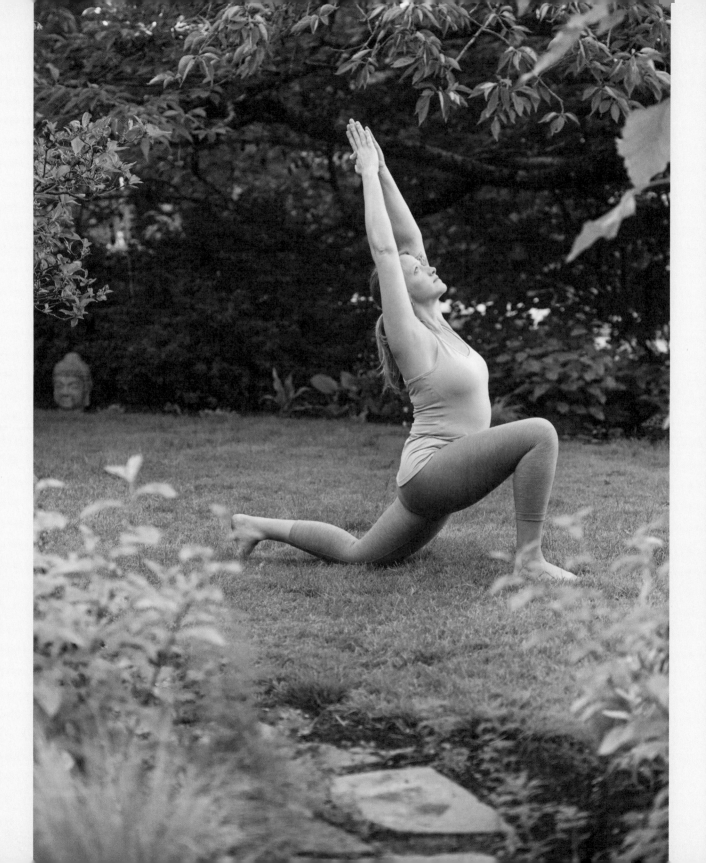

Your Body as Sanctuary

CARING FOR YOUR PERSONAL ECOSYSTEM

Our body is our soul's temple, and its needs must be honored for us to achieve our highest potential.

The spaces we spend the most time in can and should be treated as sacred. There is no other space we spend more time in than our body—our soul's temple, our only vehicle in life. Yet we don't always make choices that are healthy for it. We are not taught to make self-care a priority. We live in a culture with physical and mental struggles: obesity, diabetes, cancer, heart disease, depression, and anxiety disorders, to name a few. If we are looking to find sanctuary in our lives, it is important to look at how we care for ourselves. Our body is an intelligent biological organism, and we have the ability to listen to our body's wisdom if we choose to.

What if we looked at our body as we do a plant? Plants have ideal growing conditions, hormonal responses, and genetic potential. We too have ideal growing conditions and hormonal responses, and we can reach our highest genetic potential if we choose to. What are our ideal growing conditions? I like to use this line

of thinking as a way to filter out what isn't needed in my life. We need clean water and pure food, healthy ways to move our bodies, ways to relax and pamper ourselves, and plenty of restful sleep. With the aid of the sanctuary you have created and the plant allies you have cultivated there, you can make these vital nutrients part of your personal ecosystem.

Detoxing from Modern Life

Just by taking part in everyday life, our bodies absorb toxins—from air pollution, from the water we drink and bathe in, from chemically treated food, and from products we use. For instance, one of every three chemical cleaning products contains ingredients known to cause human health or environmental problems, and the most common source of exposure to poisons for children under age six is cosmetics / personal care

159

products, according to the 2006 Annual Report of the American Association of Poison Control Centers' National Poison Data System. When I found out that my own city's water supply contains six contaminants at levels above those established as safe by government health authorities, I began to research water filters and detox methods. You can find out more about your own city's water supply and filters to use by visiting the Environmental Working Group's Tap Water Database at ewg.org/tapwater.

With detoxes of every kind on the market these days, it isn't hard to find cleansing packages to buy. While these may have some merit, you really need look no farther than your healing garden for help. A necessary first step is to clear your fridge and pantry of any and all processed foods and beverages. Rule: if the food has an ingredient you don't know or can't pronounce the name of, it goes. Then clear your bathroom of any products with unnatural or chemical-based ingredients. You can turn to your garden for foods, drinks, and cleaning products that are much better for your personal ecosystem.

FLAVORED WATERS FOR HEALTHY HYDRATION

Start by thinking about water. Our bodies are made up of 60 to 80 percent water, and drinking more water, preferably filtered, helps with digestion, headaches, fatigue, and other symptoms of dehydration. If you replace sodas and other sugary high-calorie drinks with water, your body will thank you with better health. But drinking plain water can sometimes get boring. Water infused with fruits and herbs is appealing to the senses and enjoyable to create. It has the added benefits of providing nutrients and flushing toxins from your body.

The basic procedure is to put fruit and/or herbs in the bottom of a 2-quart mason jar or pitcher, smash it gently with the handle of a wooden spoon to release some of the juices, fill to the top with filtered water, and stir. You can keep one or several jars or pitchers lidded in the fridge for up to three days. I like to use whatever fruits and herbs are on hand and in season. You can use just about any ripe fruit except for bananas; berries from bushes in

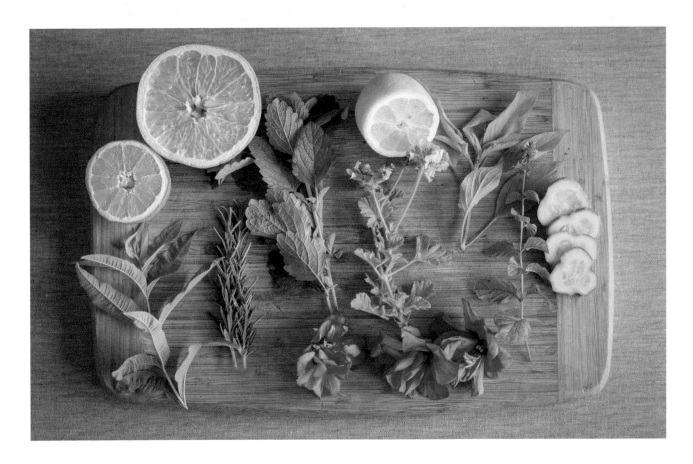

You can use fruits, vegetables, herbs, and flowers from the garden to infuse plain drinking water with flavor.

your garden are ideal. Citrus, pineapple, and watermelon are also good choices. Many herbs are a surprising complement to fruit flavors. A few of my favorites are mint, lemon balm, rosemary, and basil.

Here are some combinations to try:

* blueberry and lemon balm

* strawberry and basil

* cucumber and lemon

* apple and cinnamon sticks

* watermelon, orange, and lemon grass

* ginger and mango

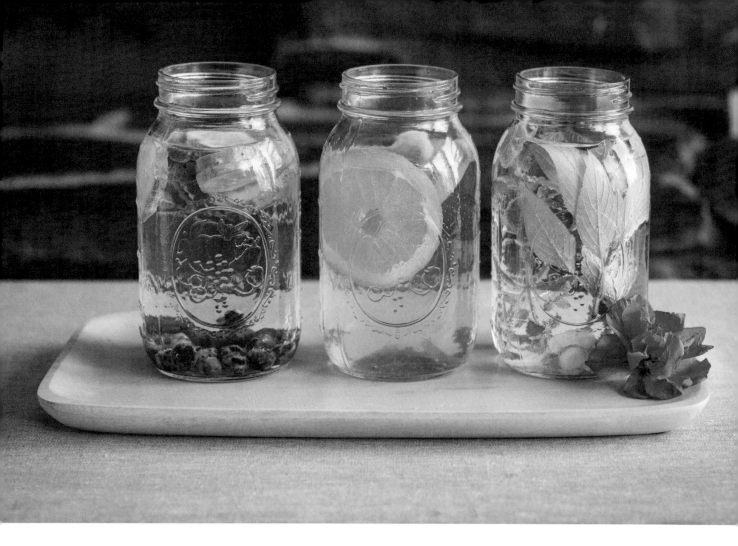

Raspberry-Lime-Mint Flavored Water

Experiment with different combinations to find out what tastes best to you.

This water has a beautiful color and is mildly tart. It provides vitamin C as well as aiding digestion.

2 limes
½ cup raspberries
a handful of mint leaves

Wash the skin of the limes well, then quarter the limes and squeeze the juice into the jar with your hands. Throw the lime quarters in and add the raspberries and mint. Press and twist with the handle of a wooden spoon just enough to release some juices but not pulverize the fruit and mint. Add ice if desired and then fill to the top with filtered water. Stir, cover, and refrigerate.

HERBS TO LOOSEN THE GRIP OF ADDICTIONS

The most common of human vices involve powerful plant products that alter the human psyche—with nicotine, alcohol, and caffeine at the top of this list. Though all have benefits, they can also become more destructive than beneficial. There are herbs that can help wean us off plants we have developed an unhealthy relationship with. These plant allies help with nicotine addiction: California poppy, ginseng, lobelia, marshmallow, oat, peppermint, slippery elm, St. John's wort, and valerian. Treat an alcohol hangover with chicory, ginger, milk thistle, peppermint, or turmeric. If you want to wean yourself off coffee, roasted root tea makes a great substitute.

Roasted Root Tea

FOR 1 QUART OF BEVERAGE:
2 teaspoons roasted chicory root
2 teaspoons roasted dandelion root
ashwagandha root or eleuthero root (optional)
1 quart of hot water

Place the chicory and dandelion roots in a French press or coffeemaker. Allow to steep in the hot water for four to six minutes before pouring. Add milk, sweetener, or other ingredients as desired—I like mine with cinnamon and almond milk, or you can try orange peel and/or cardamom.

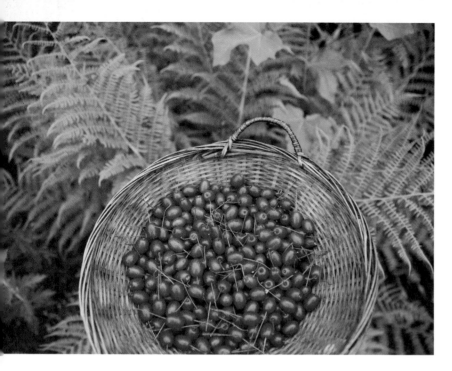

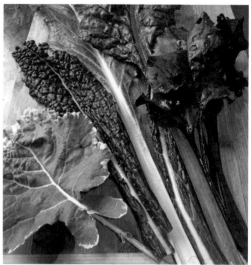

Goumi berries grow on attractive nitrogen-fixing shrubs and are full of vitamin C, lycopene, and antioxidants.

ABOVE RIGHT Swiss chard, kale, and collard greens are easy to grow in a healing garden and are among the superfoods that boost health.

Garden Nutrition and Mindful Meals

Foods like berries, vegetables, and nuts that are packed with nutrients and contain higher levels of antioxidants, vitamins, and minerals than other plants are known as superfoods. Unprocessed and straight from the earth, these are the foods we are biologically designed to eat. They can help us fight disease, feel more energetic, and even lose weight. You can buy these at the grocery store, but you will be more confident that they were grown without chemicals and you will have a stronger connection to them if you grow them at home. This is in line with what is known in Ayurveda as the sattvic diet, which is vegetarian and emphasizes foods richest in prana or life

force energy—fresh, organic, whole foods, grown and prepared with care.

Here are some easy-to-grow superfoods, by plant layer:

* trees—almonds, apples, cherries, mulberries, plums, walnuts

* shrubs—aronia, blueberries, goji, goumi, green tea, raspberries

* herbaceous perennials—asparagus, artichokes, fuki, horseradish, rhubarb

* ground layer—garlic, oca, potatoes, pumpkins/squash, strawberries, yacon

* climbers—beans, climbing yams, grapes, kiwis, nasturtiums, passionflower

* annuals—arugula, beets, broccoli, greens (kale, collard greens, chard, spinach), turnips, sunflowers

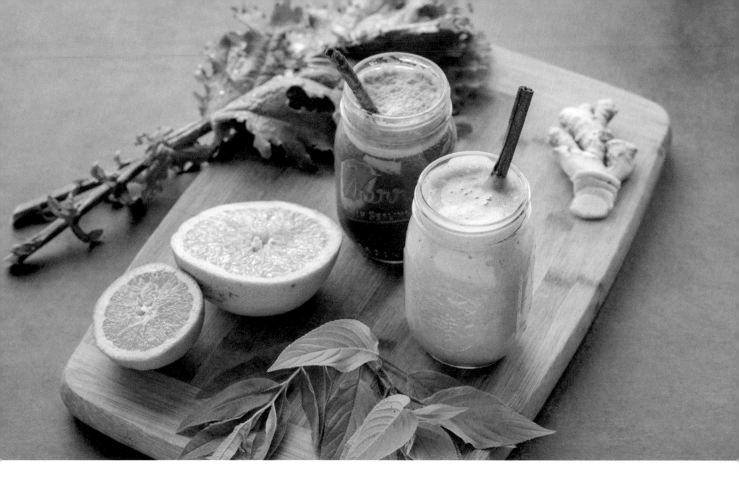

Garden Smoothie

An easy way to get a quick dose of nourishment is to blend superfoods fresh from the garden into a smoothie. A high-quality blender is a necessity and has become a cherished kitchen appliance at my house.

a handful of leafy greens (spring greens, lettuce, chard, kale, spinach, parsley)

a handful of fruit (berries, banana, apple, pineapple, orange, pear, grapes)

optional yogurt, protein powder, herbs, and/or spices (ginger, lemon verbena, mint, cinnamon, or others)

enough liquid to cover (water, coconut water, fruit juice, unsweetened almond or coconut milk)

Add ingredients, blend, and drink (smoothies don't make good leftovers).

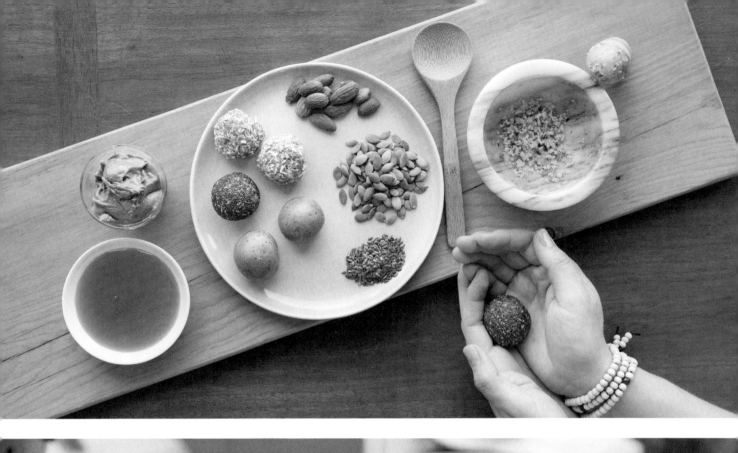

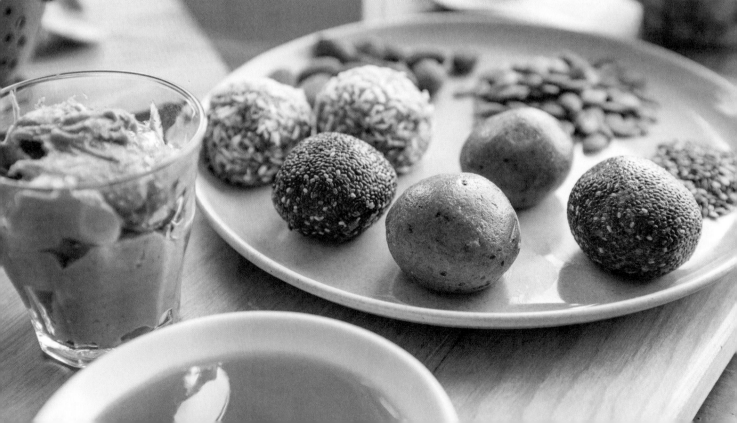

Protein Bombs

Protein bombs made with honey, nut butter, almonds, pumpkin seeds, flax seeds, and crushed walnuts are a quick on-the-go snack.

Also on the list of superfoods are nut butters and seeds. Nuts and seeds are not as easy to harvest and process but can be purchased and made into powerhouse snacks for a quick pick-me-up when you are on the go. You can vary the ingredients to use what you have on hand or just to be creative.

½ cup nuts (walnuts, almonds,
   macadamias, pistachios)
½ cup nut butter (peanut, almond, cashew)
½ cup seeds (sunflower, chia, hemp,
   flax, pumpkin, sesame)
¼ cup dried fruit (raisins, cranberries,
   goji berries, apricots, cherries)
½ teaspoon spices (cinnamon,
   cardamom, cloves, nutmeg)
optional ingredients: oats, protein
   powder, matcha, chocolate chips,
   coconut flakes, vanilla
enough honey, maple syrup, and/or
   mashed banana to hold things together

Mix your chosen ingredients together in a bowl until everything adheres and can be formed into balls. Using your hands, shape the mixture into balls a little smaller than a golf ball. Place in a container and refrigerate to eat later. Depending on the ingredients used, you can keep them in the fridge for about a week, or in the freezer for longer.

Herbs to help digestion

Much of our well-being is related to gut health. If we don't keep our digestive tract in balance, whether as a result of stress or eating something that doesn't agree with our system, we can be subject to a variety of ailments or painful symptoms. Many plants can help us keep our digestive system healthy. Before we eat, taking *bitters* from plant allies including mugwort, yarrow, calendula, and dandelion can help us produce enzymes and secretions to help stimulate our system. Fennel can warm up the digestive tract and help rid us of gas and cramping. *Demucilants* including marshmallow, slippery elm, aloe, and licorice help coat the mucus membrane of the digestive tract and ease heartburn, inflammation, ulcers, constipation, and irritable bowel syndrome.

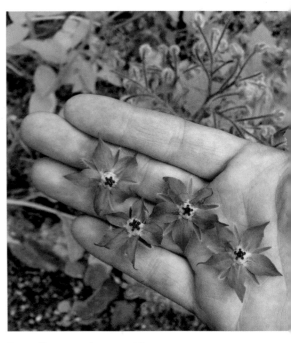

Borage flowers used as a garnish can dress up a salad or a soup.

As important as what you eat is how you eat it. Meals are about much more than just food—they are about our connection to the earth and the people around us. In cultures around the world, sharing a meal with others has been a longtime ritual to create togetherness and bonding. Providing nourishment for yourself and others can be a celebration, from the harvesting to the preparation to the eating. Even if you eat alone, you can create a meaningful experience by eating mindfully, conscious of what went into every bite, the seed and the sun and the rain and the soil, the farmer if it was someone other than you. Eating slowly is also a good habit, since our mind doesn't tell us we are satiated until about twenty minutes after our stomach is full.

Your backyard sanctuary can be a lovely setting for meals if you pay some attention to providing space for it. You might also pay special attention to presenting foods from the garden attractively. Herbs and flowers such as borage and nasturtium petals look beautiful garnishing soups and salads. Leaves, branches, and flowers can be used to decorate the table.

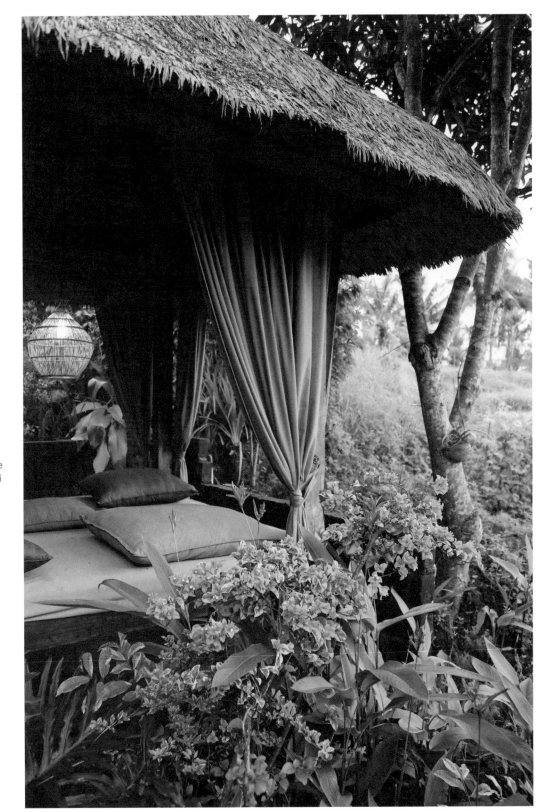

This relaxing space at the edge of a rice field in Bali makes a lovely setting for a simple meal.

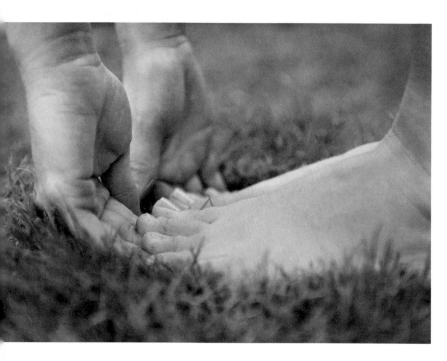

Basic stretching is one of the best daily body care habits we can adopt.

Mindful Movement

Our bodies love to move. Let's face it—we are not designed to sit in chairs or drive in cars; we are designed to be active, walk, squat, carry things, and move our bodies. Our bodies are *built* to move, and many of us don't move nearly enough. Tending your personal sanctuary—whether watering plants or trimming and pruning, weeding, planting, hauling compost and mulch, or harvesting fresh vegetables and herbs—is one enjoyable way to get your body in motion while building your relationship with your plant allies.

During this workout, be mindful of your body's fascia. Fascia is the connective tissue throughout our bodies that holds together, attaches, separates, and encloses all structures: organs and other tissues like ligaments and muscles. I think of it as a big fibrous spiderweb-like layer of our inner skin. This tissue is responsible for our body's stabilization and movement. To care for your fascia, you need to stay hydrated and to stretch. Take five minutes to do some easy stretches outside in the fresh air before exerting yourself in the garden. Breathe in and out slowly and deeply, and stretch only as far as you comfortably can. Stop and stretch periodically while you are gardening, too.

Your personal sanctuary is also an ideal place to practice yoga, tai chi, qigong, and/or mindful walking. These ancient arts aim to create harmony in our body and mind and can be practiced by anyone. When you practice them outdoors, there is an additional benefit. A variety of scientific studies have confirmed what we already know in our bones, that when we spend time in nature, we feel better. "Green exercise improves psychological health," says Richard Louv, whose book *The Nature Principle* is a good summary of this research. Spending time outdoors in mindful movement can relax and ground your nervous system.

A space for your movement practice can be as simple as a lawn or a deck. To create the right ambience, you can use some of the sacred space elements we discussed earlier, such as altars, cairns, prayer flags, garden art, and water features. You might keep your yoga mat or

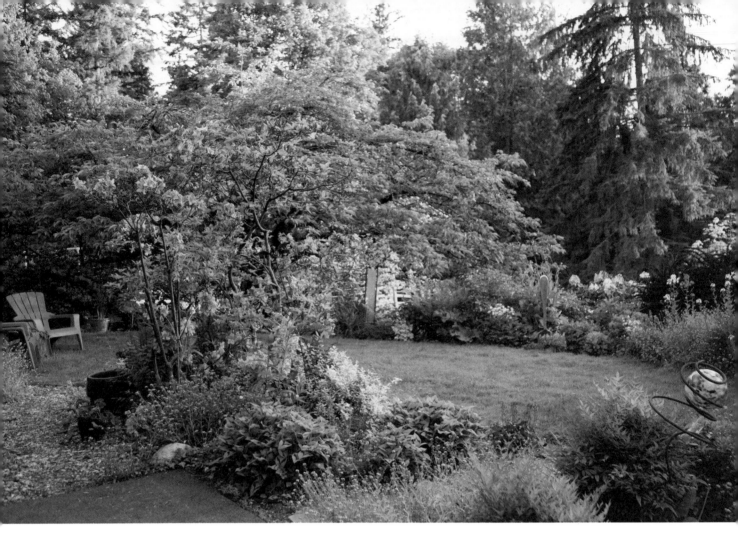

My outdoor space for mindful movement includes garden art and blooming plants.

towel by the back door ready to use in this area, and you could provide a place to leave shoes. My outdoor movement space has a statue, some art, and colorful and fragrant blooming plants throughout the growing season.

You can also bring the quality of reverence for your body to your practice. Think of bathing your whole body in the reverence you would feel while sitting at the foot of a great tree or standing at the bottom of a wild waterfall. As you engage in the form of mindful movement of your choice, listen closely to your body to notice its needs and imagine how you can fill them with connection to the beauty of nature in your sanctuary.

Nothing says that any of these movement practices need to be done in segments of any particular length to be effective, so I suggest picking one of these practices and doing it for just a few minutes in your sanctuary every day if you don't have time for more. Doing some of the

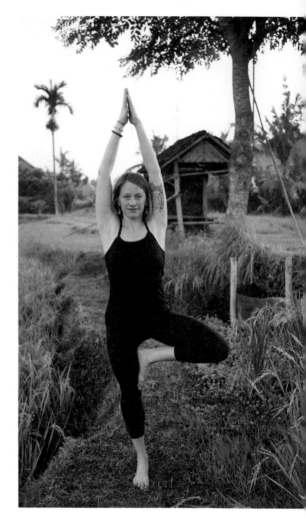

Tree pose (vrksasana) takes on an added dimension when practiced in a sanctuary space outdoors.

practices outdoors may not be practical during the winter months but you can at least do them outdoors during the summer.

YOGA

Yoga originated in ancient India and is currently practiced by close to 10 percent of the world's population. It emphasizes clearing the way for *prana*, the Sanskrit word for life energy, to circulate freely throughout our bodies. It includes physical postures to improve flexibility, strength, focus, and balance, as well as breathing exercises to help us relax and center ourselves. Western science has been studying the neurological and physical benefits of yoga, and has found that regular practice can significantly reduce negative emotional states and improve our immune response to stressors. For some it begins as a way to heal from physical stress and evolves to become a spiritual practice and a way to develop mind-body awareness.

If you don't already practice yoga but want to try it, I suggest taking a few classes and getting guidance from a teacher as you start out. Yoga classes at all levels are becoming more and more commonly available wherever you may live. I've had a variety of teachers and practice both in studios and at home. When the weather permits, I do yoga outdoors and find that the fresh air, fragrances, sounds, and sights all help to ground me. I pay particular attention to visualizing a connection to the earth while doing the poses. For instance, seeing myself as a tree helps me to find strength and stability while in tree pose; I imagine myself growing roots from the base of my spine extending into the ground and reaching the center of the earth.

Herbs to relax sore muscles

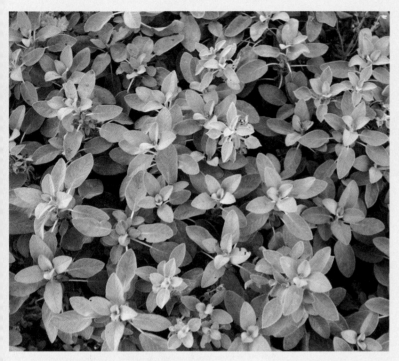

Sage, known for its anti-inflammatory properties, can help ease sore muscles.

As someone who is active will attest, using your body means you will feel it—all over. Sometimes you will have sore muscles or tight tissues from a physical workout like gardening or yoga. Plant allies can help you with this. Hyssop and marshmallow root in tea soothes inflammation, while chamomile tea can aid relaxation. Skullcap, sage, and turmeric in tea can ease muscle pain, and peppermint or lemongrass in a tea or compress helps relax cramping and tight muscles. Cayenne pepper and meadowsweet in creams can relieve pain.

QIGONG AND TAI CHI

Qigong (pronounced "chee gung") has been called Chinese yoga. It is an ancient Chinese practice (going back five thousand years) that seeks to cultivate qi or chi, the body's life force energy, through meditative movement. Tai chi originated in Taoist qigong and is similar in many ways. Both use slow, flowing movements done mostly in a standing position, deep breathing, and visualization to improve the health and harmony of mind and body. Both are commonly practiced outdoors. Experimental evidence suggests that qigong practice lowers the resting heart rate, improves circulation, improves blood flow to the brain, improves posture and balance, reduces pain, alleviates anxiety and depression, and improves the immune system and longevity.

There are more than sixty-five hundred qigong moves, with names as enchanting and suggestive as Hands Waving Clouds and Calming the Waters. Find a video online or a local teacher and try it out if you aren't already a practitioner. Whether you are just beginning or experienced, focus on the benefits of having your feet planted on the earth while you do it in your personal sanctuary.

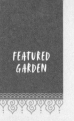
THE ZEN MAYOR'S GARDEN

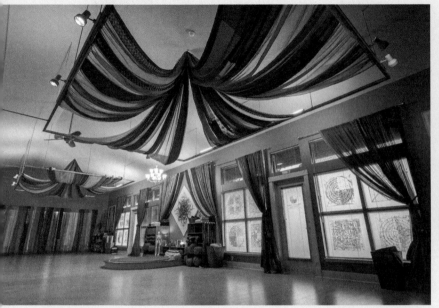

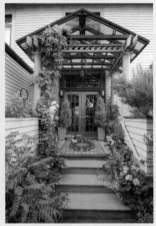

AngelArmsWorks is a welcoming space for art and community.

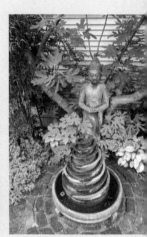

A fig tree provides a backdrop for Karen's own garden of Eden.

Karen's yoga studio was the first in Snohomish, Washington.

KAREN GUZAK IS AN ARTIST AND A YOGI who served as mayor of Snohomish, Washington, for eight years—a truly inspirational and remarkable woman. A lifelong artist, she has made her home and garden a sacred space for art and community. She purchased a run-down historic (1889) church building at auction in 1990, and with her partner, Warner Blake, devoted nearly ten years to restoring it into a multifunctional community space. Dubbed AngelArmsWorks, it is now her and Warner's home as well as a gathering place often filled with celebrations, live music, and creating art.

Karen discovered yoga when she was fifty and quickly became a passionate yogi. In 2003 she opened Yoga Circle Studio, the first yoga studio in Snohomish, a fast-growing rural community northeast of Seattle along Puget Sound. She realized as she watched the "garden of Eden" being bombed in Iraq during the George W. Bush administration that she could make a difference by building her own garden of Eden at home. She served as mayor of Snohomish from 2009 to 2017, a reflection of her feeling that "I want to have my life count for something. I want to make a positive impact in some way. To make a difference."

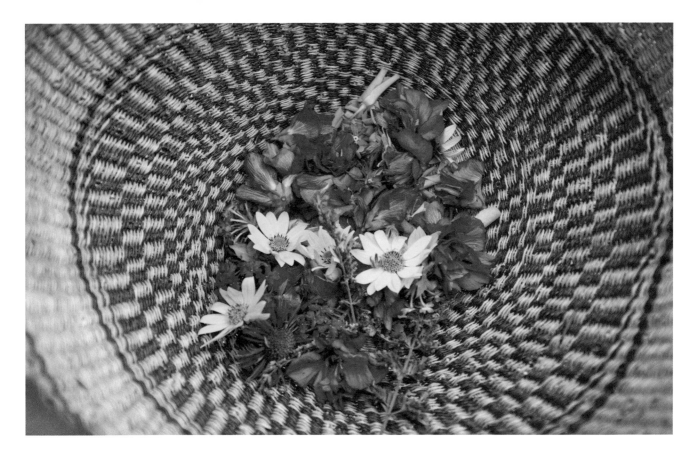

Spa Time: Self-Care Rituals

Gathering flowers and herbs for self-care rituals can help keep you connected to the garden.

Scheduling time to pamper ourselves is probably the most important thing we can do to stay healthy. This is especially crucial in a hectic life with a lot of demands and not much free time. Bathing and cleansing our bodies is one of the best opportunities to create intentional rituals for self-care and really practice loving and recentering ourselves. We can use flowers and herbs freshly harvested from our sacred garden to bring indoors the powerful benefits of the sanctuary we are cultivating.

Water is incredibly healing. Taking a bath or shower can be cleansing, renewing, relaxing, and uplifting for your body, mind, and spirit. All day long, we are in contact with energy from people around us, and this can often take us away from ourselves. Spending time alone soaking in or being rinsed by water can help us reconnect with ourselves. Warm water's naturally relaxing qualities can be enhanced by pouring a strong herbal tea into the water. Some of the tea's medicinal components will be absorbed through your skin, and some will rise into your nostrils with the steam and be absorbed there.

RITUAL
SPIRIT BATH

Drawing hot water into a tub full of carefully chosen plants and minerals can be a potent healing ritual. We can create specific recipes to provide just what we need at the moment—whether a medicinal bath for skin issues, a soothing bath for sore muscles, a relaxing bath to get us ready for sound sleep, or an emotionally healing bath to ease the heart. My spirit bath ritual happens at least once a week, and on several other significant dates surrounding the moon and my menstrual cycle.

Tune into how you are feeling and what you need. Light some candles, put on some music, and choose the ingredients for your bath. Here are some possibilities:

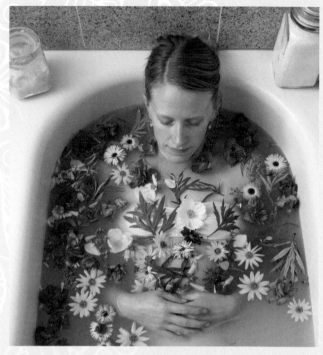

Soaking in a hot bath that incorporates carefully chosen plants and minerals can help us relax and reconnect with ourselves.

FRESH OR DRIED FLOWERS AND PLANT TISSUES
for various medical or spiritual uses.

ESSENTIAL OILS
(a few drops per bath)—to provide fragrance and specific healing effects. My top four are lavender, eucalyptus, rose, and citrus.

EPSOM SALT
(1 to 2 cups per bath)—to relax sore muscles and joints, and increase circulation.

APPLE CIDER VINEGAR
(2 cups per bath)—to balance skin pH, sooth irritations, and deodorize.

BAKING SODA
(¼ to ½ cup per bath)—to cleanse, soften, and detoxify.

OATMEAL
(1 cup ground to a powder in a blender or coffee grinder)—to soothe and soften itchy or irritated skin.

MILK
(2 cups per bath)—to hydrate, loosen dead skin, and calm irritated skin.

Draw the bath and add the ingredients. Soak for at least twenty minutes, more if you can. An inflatable pillow makes this even more relaxing.

BATH ROCK SELF-MASSAGE

While you take a bath is an excellent time to practice self-massage and focus on the areas of your body that need attention.

·1·

In your garden, find a couple of stones that fit into the palm of your hand. One should be smooth and one should have a rough texture.

·2·

Pour a bath and soak for at least twenty minutes. Then pick up the rough stone and use it to exfoliate areas of thick or dry skin such as elbows and callused feet.

·3·

Use the smooth stone to help release the tension stored in your body. Apply gentle pressure anywhere the tissue feels tense—the arches of your feet, your calves, your thighs, your lower and upper back, your neck, your arms, the palms of your hands. Work slowly with the "grain." Your limbs will appreciate long strokes, and your joints a more concentrated pressure and release. **You can do this outside of the bath as well. Warm up your stones by putting them in hot water, test the temperature for your comfort, and then use a homemade massage oil blend for lubrication.**

FOOT SOAK

Giving your feet a minibath can help you relax when you don't have time for a full bath. Simply draw hot water into a large bowl and select from the ingredients you would use for a bath.

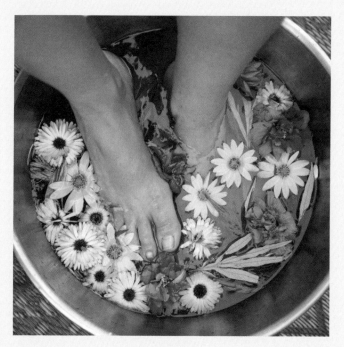

A foot soak is a small luxury you can indulge in when you don't have time for a bath.

Body Care and Home Cleaning Solutions from the Garden

Only a small percentage of chemicals in beauty products are tested for safety, and the Environmental Working Group tells us that the average woman in the United States uses twelve personal care products and/or cosmetics a day, containing 168 different chemicals. The first time I had a chemical reaction to a beauty product, it caused a painful rash on my face around my eyes. The dermatologist told me it happens all the time and I should discontinue using the product. I stopped using store-bought products at that time and began a quest to use only natural or homemade products. I discovered you can make many hair and skin care solutions and household cleansers from plants you grow in your sanctuary garden.

Making and using herbal body scrubs is a wonderful way to pamper yourself. They leave your skin feeling fresh and tingly, and they have an aromatherapy effect on your mood. Scrubs are fun to make and generally consist of an oil base (which can be infused with fresh or dried herbs of your choice), salt or sugar, and essential oils. After you make a scrub, you can store the unused portion in a glass jar in the refrigerator. Don't use a scrub more than once a week, because they have a deep exfoliating effect.

Basic Sugar or Salt Scrub

½ cup light oil such as grapeseed or almond, infused with herbs of your choice
1 cup sugar (preferably organic and raw) or salt (the coarser it is, the more exfoliating)
15 drops essential oil to match the mood you are trying to create

In a small bowl, mix the oil, sugar or salt, and essential oil together. Spoon into a sealable glass jar for use during your next spa time. Makes enough for about three uses.

You can also make hair rinses, facial toners, and home cleansers. These cost a whole lot less than you would pay at the store, and they're a whole lot better for you. Plus the process of making them will bring you in closer touch with your garden and can be a good way to spend a relaxing weekend afternoon.

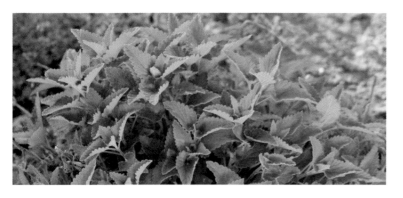

Catnip can be an effective treatment for dandruff.

Hair Rinse

Place a handful (about a cup) of freshly harvested herbs in a saucepan with four cups of water, bring to a boil, turn off the heat, and steep for twenty minutes; then strain out the herbs and apply to your hair. Here are some herbs to use:

calendula—for blond to auburn hair

catnip—for dandruff

chamomile—for blond hair

comfrey—for thinning hair, to soften and strengthen

horsetail—for oily hair and to strengthen

lavender—for dandruff, itchiness, and oily scalp

mint—for thinning hair, to soothe and invigorate

nettles—for oily hair and a flaky scalp

rosemary—for dark or thinning hair, to add shine

sage—for dark or thinning hair

Facial Toner

Place a handful (about a cup) of freshly harvested herbs in a saucepan with four cups of water, bring to a boil, turn off the heat, and steep for twenty minutes; then strain out the herbs and pat on your face. Choose from these herbs or others:

basil—for blemishes

elderflower—for oily skin

fennel—for dry skin

parsley—for acne

rose petals—for sensitive skin

witch hazel—for dry and irritated skin

Home Cleanser

Stuff a handful (a loose cup) of pine needles into a quart glass container, then fill it with cider vinegar and seal for several weeks. Dip a cloth into the solution and clean away.

Loving Touch

Touch is among the most healing and powerful ways we can bond or connect with others. Massage can be done with any willing and consenting partner, whether infants and children, pets, or significant others. Use infused oils you have prepared from your garden if you can. Children often benefit from massage before bed; using a soothing chamomile or lavender oil helps relax them for a good night's sleep. Rubbing someone's shoulders is almost a sure way to help relieve tension, and a foot rub is calming and helps the person be more grounded. In a romantic partnership, massage using oils and plants that have aphrodisiac properties (including basil, fennel, and mint) can spice things up quickly.

Learning massage can seem daunting, but you can start gently in areas that are commonly tense and easy to work on, such as the upper back and the feet. Always begin by taking some deep, cleansing breaths and imagining yourself growing roots from the base of your spine down into the earth to ground yourself. I imagine that the pressure I am applying and the motions of my hands are helping to move energy into stuck tissues and open them up. Personally, I enjoy lying on the floor on my stomach and having my partner's foot apply gentle pressure from my shoulders all the way down to my calves. This takes trust, practice, and patience but pays off both for your body and your connection with the person you are working with. If you want to know more, there are many books, classes, and professionals to check out.

Sound Sleep

Taking a hot bath with relaxing herbs, inhaling a calming essential oil such as lavender or chamomile, or drinking a tea made with herbs such as valerian and chamomile can help us prepare for restful sleep. Herbal pillows that can be warmed over and over again (in the microwave, on a radiator, or in front of the fireplace) can also alleviate stress, soothe sore muscles, help us have more vivid and memorable dreams, and protect us from nightmares.

Bedtime Bath Tea

½ cup fresh or ¼ cup dried
   chamomile flowers
½ cup fresh or ¼ cup dried lemon
   balm or peppermint leaf
¼ cup fresh or 2 tablespoons
   dried lavender flowers
several drops essential oil of your choice

Put the herbs into a sock or cloth pouch and add a few drops of essential oil. Tie off the top to make a sachet, and hang it under the tub waterspout so the hot water goes through the herbs as you draw your bath. Then just let the bag float in your bath and squeeze water through it a few times to infuse the water with herbal essence. You can prepare this tea ahead of time as well and pour into the tub, then float the sachet while you're soaking.

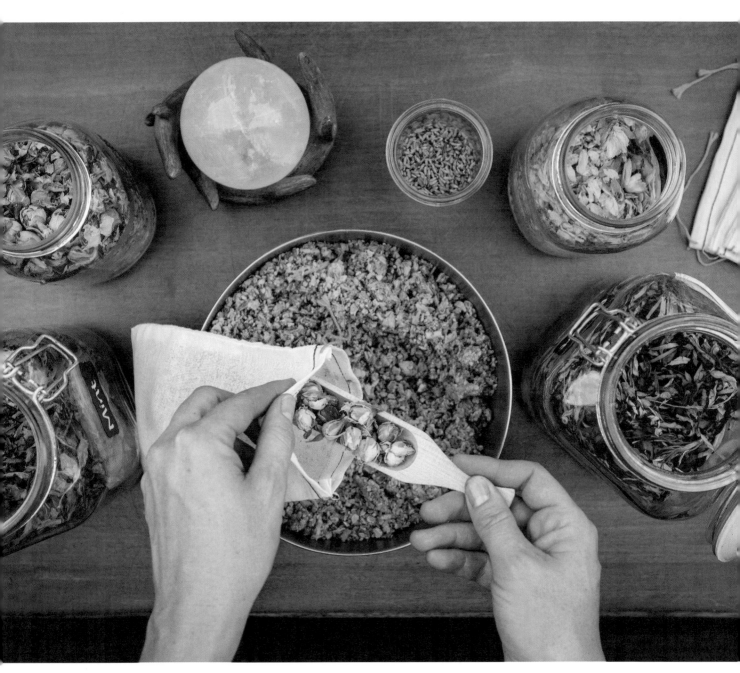

A dream pillow can be
filled with a variety of
dried herbs to pro-
mote restful sleep.

Herbal Dream Pillow

small sealable pouch (hand sewn
   or purchased) no larger than 5 by
   8 inches, or an old sock
stuffing: flax seeds, rice, or beans
a handful of dried herbs of your choice

These herbs are frequently used in dream pillows:

catnip—relaxing

chamomile—calming

hops—healing and calming

lavender—calming and relaxing

lemon balm—sedative, protects against nightmares

lemongrass—exotic, invites vivid dreams

marjoram—calming, helps with anxiety

mugwort—protective, produces lucid and prophetic dreaming

mullein—protects against nightmares

peppermint—invites vivid and prophetic dreams

rose petals—invites loving dreams

sage—promotes peaceful and healing dreams

Add your favorite herbal ingredients to the pouch or sock (experiment with different blends for different uses), fill with stuffing, and seal. Warm it up to release the fragrance and take a deep whiff of it before sleep. Do not wash.

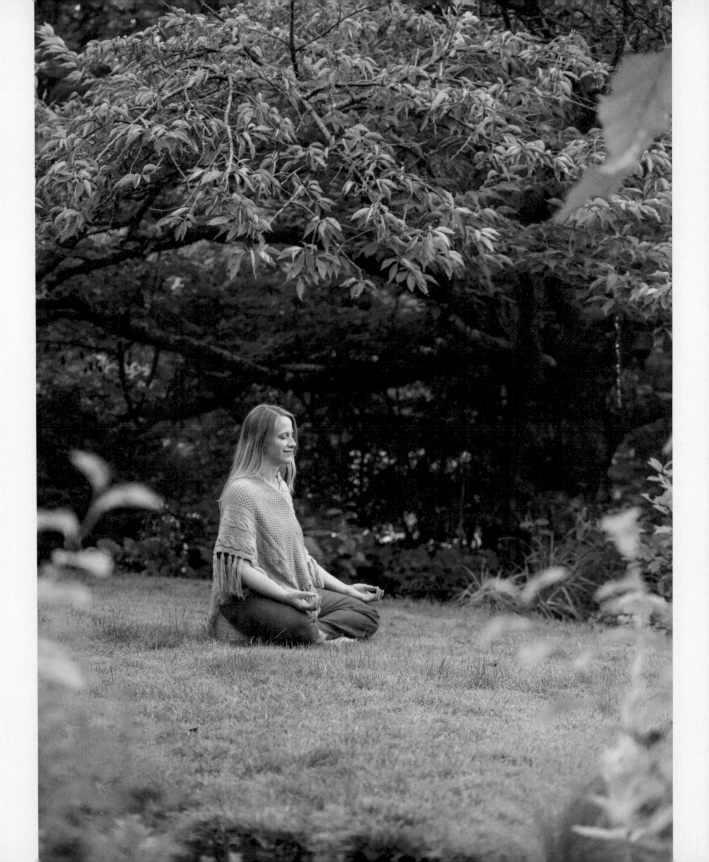

Mind and Soul

FINDING CLARITY AND COMFORT

Time spent meditating in your sanctuary can help you find clarity and comfort.

When we begin taking better care of our bodies by using our sanctuary space to connect with nature's healing benefits, we may also find our thoughts and emotions becoming more positive. Time spent close to nature is therapeutic and can help us cope with the inevitable ups and downs of life. No matter who we are, we all experience anxiety, sadness, heartbreak, grief, distress, anger, confusion, hurt, disappointment, and other challenging emotions. Our sanctuary offers many ways to work constructively with such feelings and to find soul nourishment in connections with plants, animals, and other people.

The key is to begin to see your sanctuary as a safe place to tune in to difficult emotions and fully feel them, to listen to your body and what it tells you about the impact of various emotions. Emotional intelligence is not taught in our culture as a valued skillset, yet it can be incredibly helpful in staying healthy. So can cultivating meaningful connections with yourself and others in outdoor play and ceremony, and developing a conscious relationship with nature's seasons and cycles.

Calming the Nervous System

Our bodies grow from seeds, just like plants. We share the same life force energy. And as energetic beings, we have energy running through our nervous systems every second of every minute of every day. Many cultures around the world acknowledge that keeping that life force energy connected to the earth is at the core of health. Much like a house with an electrical wiring system, we need to have our current grounded to avoid problems. Being outdoors in contact with the earth can help keep us grounded and calm our nervous system.

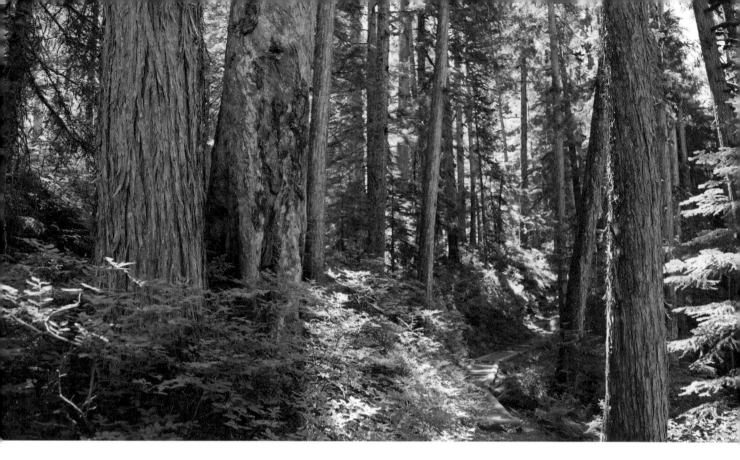

"Bathing" in the beneficial chemicals and energies emitted by plants and trees can be calming, rejuvenating, and restoring to the nervous system.

Outdoor therapy approaches have roots in many cultures throughout the ages. Sierra Club founder John Muir was an advocate, saying, "Climb the mountains and get their good tidings. Nature's peace will flow into you as sunshine flows into trees. The winds will blow their own freshness into you, and the storms their energy, while cares will drop away from you like the leaves of autumn." When stress has disrupted your equilibrium, there are a number of activities and practices you can do outdoors to bring yourself back into balance.

FOREST BATHING

In Japan and elsewhere since the 1980s, researchers have been studying the benefits of a practice called forest bathing (*shinrin yoku*). The idea is simply for a person to visit a natural area and walk in a relaxed way in order to experience calming, rejuvenating, and restorative effects. In particular, researchers have found that besides having physical benefits like lowering blood pressure and boosting immune system functioning, forest bathing improves mood, increases the ability to focus (even in children with ADHD),

GROUNDING OR EARTHING

·1·

Start by breathing deeply.

·2·

Stand or sit comfortably with both feet flat on the ground. This can work anywhere, but for the most effective experience, have your bare feet directly touching the earth if possible. You can also do this while lying down on the earth.

·3·

Next, find your feet by concentrating on feeling the soles, and wiggle your toes if that helps bring awareness to that area of your body.

·4·

Inhale deeply as you imagine bringing the raw energy of the earth into the bottoms of your feet and pulling it up your legs into your torso.

·5·

On your exhale, visualize letting all of your negative energy trickle down into your feet and drain out the bottoms through energetic roots. Let the earth take all of that stress, fear, anxiety, and trauma and compost it.

·6·

On your next inhale, imagine those roots carrying a sense of peace and nourishment up through the soles of your feet and into your body, making its way into your heart.

·7·

Repeat the inhale and exhale, exchanging energy through your feet with the earth until your roots are deep.

and increases energy levels. People who practice it regularly say that it has given them clearer intuition, increased capacity to communicate with the land and its species, and deeper friendships, as well as increasing their overall sense of happiness.

Forest bathing is a growing movement, and some resorts in the United States such as the Mohonk Mountain House in New Paltz, New York, have started to offer forest-bathing programs. Often they combine leisurely walking with guided activities, meditations, and group discussions. You can reap the benefits of forest bathing in your own backyard simply by walking slowly through your sanctuary and doing some deep breathing in the presence of your plants while being mindful of the phytoncides they are giving off. These are airborne chemicals that plants produce to protect themselves from insects. Phytoncides have antibacterial and antifungal qualities, and breathing them in is beneficial to the human immune system.

GROUNDING AND MEDITATING

One way to discharge any negative energy you may be carrying in your nervous system such as trauma, fear, anxiety, or stress is by grounding. This practice can help you feel the comfort of gravity anchoring you to the earth. Practice this whenever

MEDITATING IN NATURE

·1·

Sit comfortably with your eyes closed. You may be more comfortable sitting in a chair or with your back against the trunk of a tree.

·2·

Breathe comfortably through your nose and become aware of the sensation of your breath as it flows in and out of your nostrils.

·3·

Hold your attention on your breathing without trying to control it. If you notice your attention wandering away, simply bring it back to the breath. Do this as often as you need to, and refrain from judging yourself.

·4·

Sit in this way for ten to twenty minutes, then open your eyes.

As an alternative to keeping your attention on your breath during meditation, you can focus on your body and slowly scan it from the inside, starting at your feet and moving all the way up to the crown of your head. Or you can hold in mind this series of questions and wait for the answers to come:

PHYSICAL LAYER

Is my body healthy, or do I have illness, aches, and pains? Do I feel strong, or tired and weak?

EMOTIONAL LAYER

Have I been making decisions out of fear, anger, and shame, or have I been operating from a place of peace and happiness?

MENTAL LAYER

Do I have clear thoughts, or do I feel confused? Have I been having paranoid thoughts?

SPIRITUAL LAYER

Do I have faith in something larger than myself and trust my intuition? Or do I lack trust and belief?

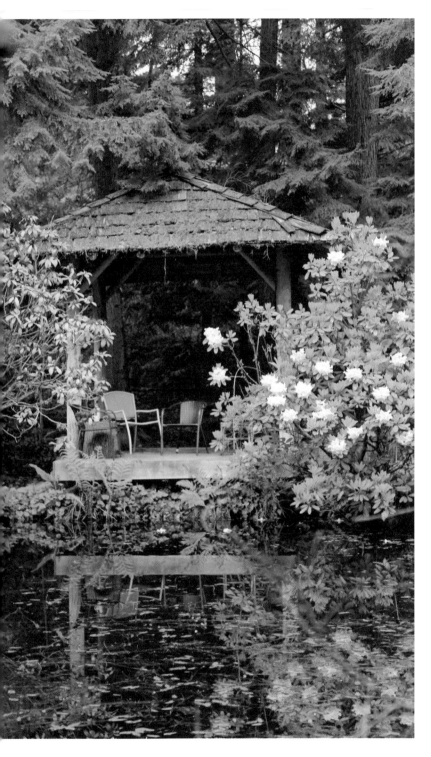

A gazebo at the edge of a quiet pond is a restful place to find solace in meditation or reflection.

you are feeling overwhelmed, upset, or stressed in any way. If you practice it enough, it will become second nature.

"Remember the entrance door to the sanctuary is inside you," advised the Persian poet Rumi. One of the easiest ways to use your sacred space for sanctuary is to meditate there, even for five minutes. There are many ways to meditate, and many beneficial reasons to do it. Meditation has been scientifically proven to reduce inflammation, increase immune function, decrease pain, lower cortisol levels, decrease ruminative thinking and anxiety, and increase happiness. Meditation takes you away from present concerns and puts you in touch with the wisdom of your body and soul, which speak to you when your mind is quiet. Meditating in nature has the added benefit of making it easier for you to focus by removing you from the distractions of other people and technology.

MEDITATION
LABYRINTH WALK

·1·

Before you enter and walk a labyrinth, it is a good idea to center and ground yourself. Stand at the entrance and find your breath. Clear your mind, letting go of your everyday thoughts, and focus on what your intentions are. If you want to find help or guidance, be clear in asking what you want to learn. I have found that it is helpful to find a word to focus on—for example, *peace* or *love* or *heal*.

·2·

As you walk, focus on your intent or just feel the space around you.

·3·

Once you reach the center, you can pause, even sit or lie down, and take time to reflect on your journey thus far.

·4·

When you are ready to walk out of the labyrinth, focus on any guidance you have received and feel gratitude.

WALKING THE LABYRINTH

If you have included a labyrinth in your sanctuary space or have access to one nearby, walking the labyrinth is a time-tested way to find clarity and calm. Give yourself the freedom to use the labyrinth in whatever way you need and to do it without a time limit. You can walk barefoot for more of a connection to the earth.

Eco Art and Play

Both therapeutic and fun, playing with the earth around us can inspire great creativity, wonder, and imagination in anyone. Whether you are looking for an activity to do with the children in your life or seeking ways to allow your inner child to come out and play, there are many ways to have a fun connection with the earth in your sanctuary space. Try any of these:

- paint rocks
- build forts
- create homes for fairies
- make outdoor altars or shrines

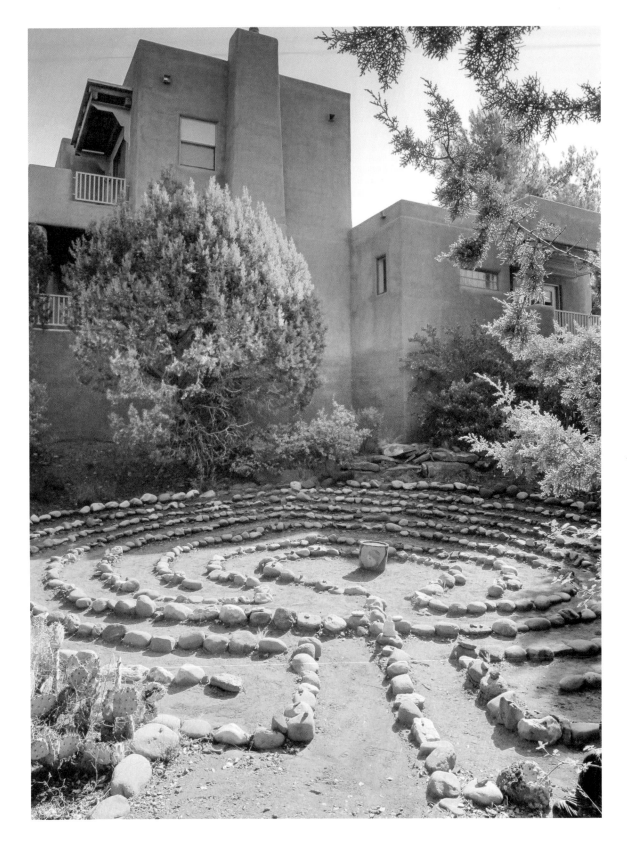

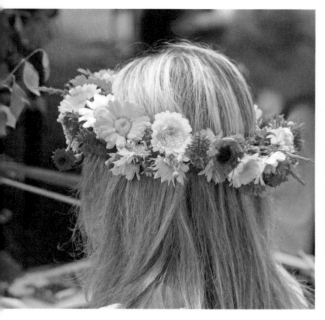

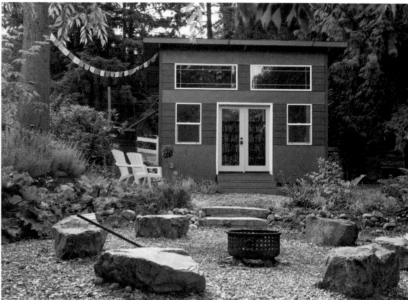

Flower crowns are easy and fun to make with plant material, a stalk of dried grass, and some twist ties.

ABOVE RIGHT This outdoor ceremony space contains seating, prayer flags, and a fire pit.

* make a mandala in the soil with collected objects

* find and collect leaf types

* carve a walking stick

* make a wreath

* make a flower or foliage bouquet

* make a flower crown

Ceremonies and Rites of Passage

Ceremonies and rituals have been a part of human life since civilization began. In the last few hundred years, though, we have lost much traditional wisdom and knowledge about rites of passage that were once essential to community building and personal growth. These days, we are largely divorced from ceremony aside from weddings and funerals. Still, the fact remains that ceremony fulfills a basic human need to mark times of transition and change.

Each of us experiences times in our life that are worth celebrating, and we also experience times that are challenging. From birth to death, we can mark birthdays, marriages, and rites of passage as well as periods of grief or mourning when a loved one dies or a relationship ends. Ultimately we all grow and change as a result of these times in our lives, but if pain is associated with the change, we may bury our feelings and move on without really acknowledging and honoring the transition. During these times, it can be very helpful to have a personal or

DESIGN YOUR OWN CEREMONY

Ceremonies can be created for a whole array of needs, whether blessing a new space, welcoming a baby, honoring a life transition, asking for our prayers to be heard, or acknowledging any other aspect of life. The basic steps are the same, no matter what the focus.

·1·

Set your intentions. Visualize or describe the outcome you desire.

·2·

Clean and clear the space. Use smudging, sound, or water to cleanse the area and yourself. Be thorough.

·3·

Call in spiritual allies for support. These can be ancestors, natural elements, religious figures, or the like.

·4·

Welcome those who are present and share intentions so that everyone feels safe.

·5·

Do activities that move energy. Singing, dancing, and chanting are especially good ways to open your heart and get energy moving through your body. Burning slips of paper on which prayers have been written, using water to bless or release objects, and using hand motions to symbolize desired results are additional ways to move energy. Use your imagination.

·6·

Wrap up with gratitude for all of the participants—people and spirits alike.

community ritual or ceremony to recognize and mark the change.

Space can be set aside for this in your outdoor sanctuary. Whether a ceremony will involve one person or a gathering of many, an altar, a space for fire, and seating are essential props. Some ceremonies require specific objects or elements, depending on the cultural lineage they are based in. I find that outdoor ceremonial spaces feel best when supported by plant allies in nearby garden beds.

In Tune with the Cycles and Seasons

The time we spend on earth is not linear but moves in cycles. Our bodies, emotions, and spirits are intimately connected to the natural rhythms of the sun, the moon, and the seasons. We enjoy better physical, mental, and spiritual health when we remember this and respect these rhythms, when we move in tune with them instead of ignoring them and pushing onward regardless, as our culture urges us to do. Cultivating sacred space in your own backyard can help you observe nature in its cycles and phases and follow its wisdom.

SOLAR AND LUNAR CYCLES

First there are the daily rhythms of the sun. Many spiritual traditions recognize

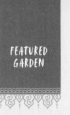

SACRED GROVES

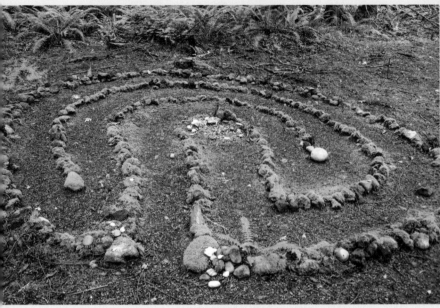

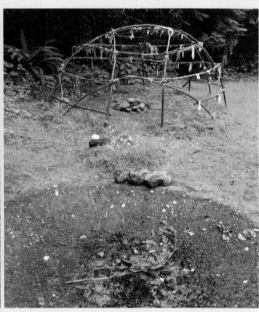

The labyrinth at Sacred Groves is a place for visitors to walk mindfully "in the healing green of the woods."

ABOVE RIGHT The ecoretreat regularly hosts sweat lodges.

SACRED GROVES is a magical 10-acre forest sanctuary on Bainbridge Island, Washington. It was created with the intention to host an ecoretreat: an artful center for music, learning, ceremonies, and rituals, and to help people heal and "open our hearts in the healing green of the woods." Founded by Thérèse Charvet in 2002 and further developed by her with Tere Carranza, this sacred space honors all walks of life and spiritualities. Between the two of them, Thérèse and Tere have a variety of skills to share: midwifery, ministry, counseling, construction, and leading ceremony with elements of ritual from spiritual lineages that connect to Mother Earth, including Buddhism, Wicca, goddess spirituality, and Native American spirituality.

Their guest lodging, Sacred Groves Bed and Breakfast, demonstrates living lightly and ecologically. They encourage forest bathing and offer classes and workshops in compassionate listening, grief support, and rites of passage, as well as spirit quests and sweat lodges. Sacred Groves truly embodies honoring the land and the diversity of all people who visit. "We welcome people from all races and cultures who share the belief that the earth is sacred and that music, dance, prayer, ceremony, and time in the natural world are essential for personal and community health."

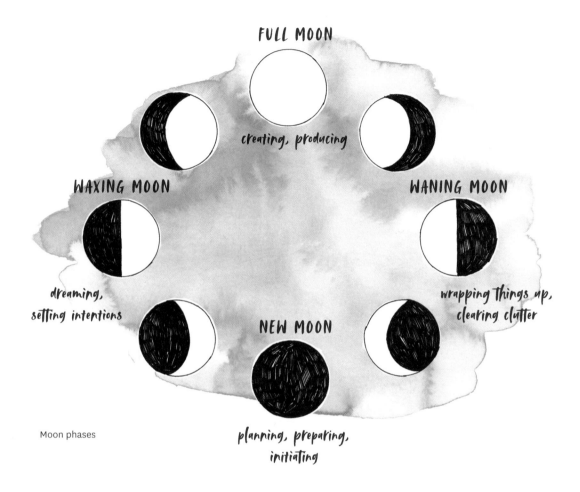

FULL MOON

creating, producing

WAXING MOON

WANING MOON

dreaming,
setting intentions

wrapping things up,
clearing clutter

NEW MOON

Moon phases

planning, preparing,
initiating

the first light of day as a powerful time, a time of shifting from dreamtime into waking life and finding your focus for the day. Greeting the rising sun in your sanctuary can be a powerful practice year-round. You can create a small ritual like stepping into the garden at first light, inhaling deeply, greeting the plants and animals, and finding a word to encapsulate your intention for the day. This is also a good time for simple stretches or yoga, or perhaps journaling about your hopes for the day. Sundown and dusk are also magical times. Stepping out into your garden for even five minutes, breathing deeply, exhaling any unwanted energies you have taken on, and expressing gratitude for all that has unfolded during your day can help settle your soul and prepare you for sleep. I find this is also a wonderful time to journal and reflect on my day and to do a simple yoga routine.

There is no denying the power of the moon. The moon rules everything

MOON FIRE CEREMONY

We can use lunar energies to help us make changes in our lives with the power of intention. Moon ceremonies can be done in your sanctuary space on the new and full moons, alone or with others. For years I have practiced this simple ritual with family and friends, and I find that even the kids like to participate.

·1·

Build a fire or just light a candle.

·2·

Clean and clear the space. Use smudging, sound, or water to cleanse the area and yourself. Be thorough.

·3·

Call in spiritual allies for support. These can be ancestors, natural elements, religious figures, or the like.

·4·

Welcome those who are present and share intentions so that everyone feels safe.

·5·

Write down an intention on a piece of paper. For the full moon, write an intention of something you want to let go of; for the new moon, an intention of something you want to receive in your life.

·6·

With others witnessing, share (aloud or silently) these intentions, and then burn them in the fire.

·7·

Close the circle with gratitude for all who attended.

◆

that flows on the earth: the ocean's tides, the life fluids in plants and animals and people, the moisture in the soil, human moods and emotions. The moon is the closest celestial body to the earth and exerts the strongest pull. Planting with the phases of the moon is an idea as old as agriculture that is based in folk wisdom but also has scientific evidence to back it up. It is said that the new moon is the best time for planting aboveground annual crops that produce seeds outside the fruit, the second quarter is the time to plant aboveground annuals with seeds inside the fruit, and after the full moon is a good time to plant root crops and perennials. By the same token, the new moon is the best time for us to plant seeds of intention with blessings for new growth; the waxing moon is a creative and expansive time full of vital energy for beginning new projects; the full moon is a time of fulfillment in projects and emotions; and the waning moon is a time for harvesting, weeding and cutting back, and preparing the ground for what comes next in your life.

THE SEASONS OF CHANGE

Each of the four seasons carries its own energy and invites us to shift our priorities and patterns to stay in alignment with what the earth is doing. Generally, spring and summer support outward activity and growth, while fall and winter encourage turning inward and resting. It can be

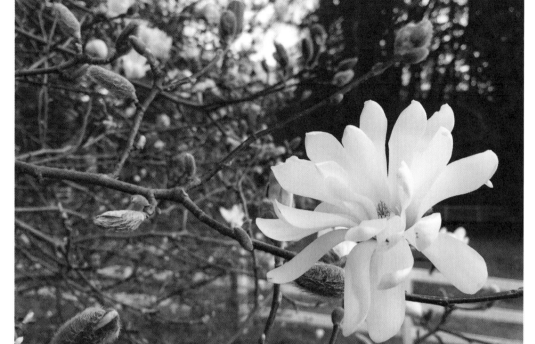

Spring calls for pushing through the darkness, opening into the light, and welcoming new energy.

a powerful centering practice to set aside time in your sanctuary on the equinoxes and solstices to reflect on the invitation of the season and how you might adapt your routines to stay in tune.

* The winter solstice on December 21 is the longest night of the year in the Northern Hemisphere. It is a time for letting go of the old year and beginning to create a vision for the new year, a time for reflecting, for going inward and seeking visions. The winter that follows is a time for resting.

* The spring equinox on March 21 marks the time when day and night

are balanced. The earth awakens at this time of inspiration and renewal. The spring season that follows is a time for planting.

* The summer solstice, June 21, marks the longest day. We are the most creative and outgoing during the summer season that follows, the season of expressing.

* The fall equinox on September 21 is again a time of equilibrium. It is a time of harvest, of gathering in energies to prepare for the colder weather and shorter days ahead. Fall is a season of emptying.

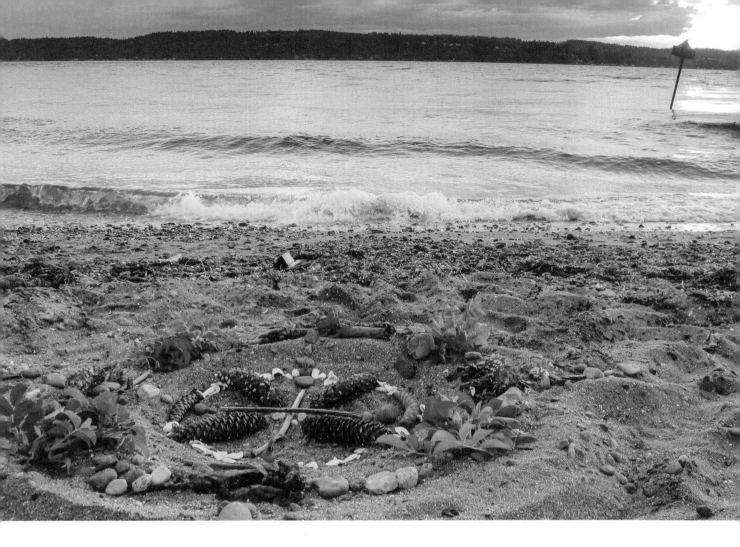

A summer solstice, or litha, flower mandala has been created on the beach.

You might write in a special journal, find an object that reminds you of the energy of the current season to place on an altar in your sanctuary space, or perform rituals, alone or with friends, on these significant days. Rituals to mark the solstices and equinoxes have been practiced by many different cultures through the ages. Summer solstice rituals, for instance, are often done at sunrise and involve prayers, or a bonfire with dancing and singing. Because my birthday lands on the summer solstice, not only do I get to celebrate my own birth but I also try to host a gathering with friends and family that involves building an altar and a mandala from plants we all have connections with. Using leaves, flowers, seeds, and stones, together we create an art piece using the four directions.

SETTING SEASONAL INTENTIONS

Writing down seasonal intentions can be a powerful practice. Consider these questions:

✳

What am I ready to let go of?

✳

What is waiting to emerge in me?

✳

What is calling for my attention deep in my soul?

✳

What quality or qualities do I want to embody in this new season?

✳

What do I want to do in this new season and what do I want to stop doing?

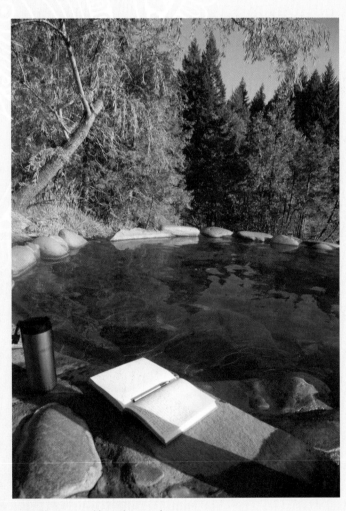

Journaling seasonal intentions can be a powerful tool for transformation.

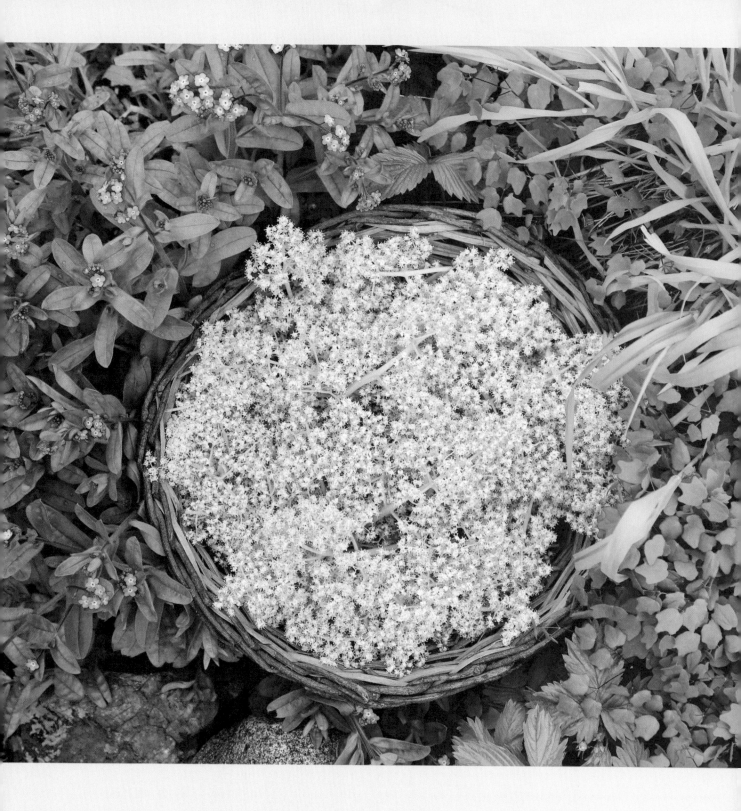

Daily Sanctuary

PRACTICES AND RITUALS

Establishing a habit of using your sanctuary every day starts with simple steps, like gathering elderberry flowers on a summer morning.

You have made a sanctuary for yourself and assembled there a variety of resources for health and well-being, including plant allies. You know how beneficial mindful movement and eating can be, along with spa time, healing touch, restful sleep, meditation, eco art and play, and ceremony. And still, the momentum of your busy life in a culture that does not encourage setting aside time for body and soul renewal may keep you from taking full advantage of what you have created and learned. You may need a new routine, new behaviors that infuse the power of sanctuary into your everyday life.

Using your sanctuary space every day and weaving the healing power of nature into your daily round doesn't need to take up a lot of your time, but it may take building new habits. A study published in 2010 in the *European Journal of Social Psychology* found that it takes anywhere from 18 to 254 days for a new

behavior to become automatic. The one thing that's certain about building a new behavior into your life is that it happens one day at a time, starting with day 1. This chapter suggests two weeks' worth of daily activities that you can do in as little as five minutes to begin to make a habit of going to your sacred space for joy, comfort, and nourishment.

Pick a time of day to do your practice, maybe first thing when you get up or after work. To get the most out of your time, unplug from everything else and let yourself be fully present. And trust that whatever time you spend, even if it's just five minutes, is beneficial. It's better to do the activity for a very short time than to skip it because you think you need more time to do it. On the other hand, if you have more time and want to extend any of these activities, go ahead. And add your own favorite activities to this list. These are just a starting place.

Day 1

MEDITATE AND JOURNAL ON YOUR VISION OF SANCTUARY

(ten minutes)

Find a comfortable place to sit, and take five minutes to read and practice the meditation exercise repeated here from the first chapter. Focus on what sanctuary means to you and how you envision the transformation in your life. Have a journal and pen nearby so that when you have finished meditating, you can write for five minutes about what you saw or felt.

Find a comfortable place to sit where you can meditate and journal for ten minutes.

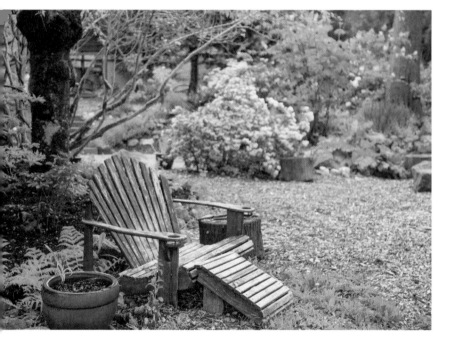

1 Get comfortable (sitting or lying down), relax, and close your eyes. Focus on taking several deep breaths and continue breathing deeply throughout the journey.

2 Start by thinking of what the word *paradise* brings up in your mind's eye. What do you see? Colors, people, plants, animals, locations, elements?

3 What do you hear? Wind, birds, talking, singing, a body of water?

4 What do you smell? Food, fragrance, plants, the weather changing?

5 What do you feel on your skin? The warmth of the sun, a gentle rain, a cool breeze?

6 What do you taste? The sweetness of fruit, the pungency of herbs?

7 What does your heart feel? Happiness, grief, joy, indifference?

8 Now open your eyes and write down what came to you.

Day 2

CREATE A PERSONAL TRANSFORMATION ALTAR

(ten to thirty minutes)

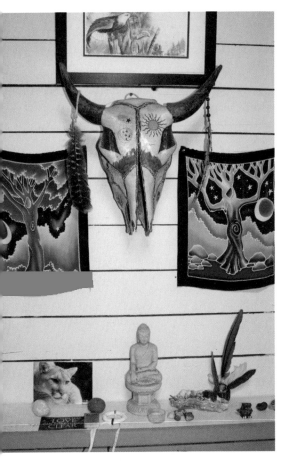

This altar for transformation was created using objects with personal meaning.

Building on your day 1 meditation and journaling, bring to mind an intention to transform something in your life. Choose a place for your altar where you'll see it often enough but it won't be in the way. Clear the space of debris, or of negative energy or thought forms, using smudging or sound bathing. Recall from earlier in the book that smudging involves burning dried plant material so that the smoke from the smoldering herbs can cleanse the area, while sound bathing is using specific sounds—such as those made by chimes, bells, singing bowls, drums, rattles, or even clapping—to change the frequency of an area.

Then place on the altar objects that have significance to you relating to your intention. Any objects you use should be cleaned both when you place them on the altar and when you remove them. I have a ritual of asking permission ("Do you want to help with this altar?") before use and always thanking the object afterward. I use items that I have collected over the years; many have been found, and some have been gifts. Sometimes I write a single word on a small piece of paper to place on my altar with a specific intention or resonance. I usually place at least four objects on the altar, considering where they might fit in with the cardinal directions.

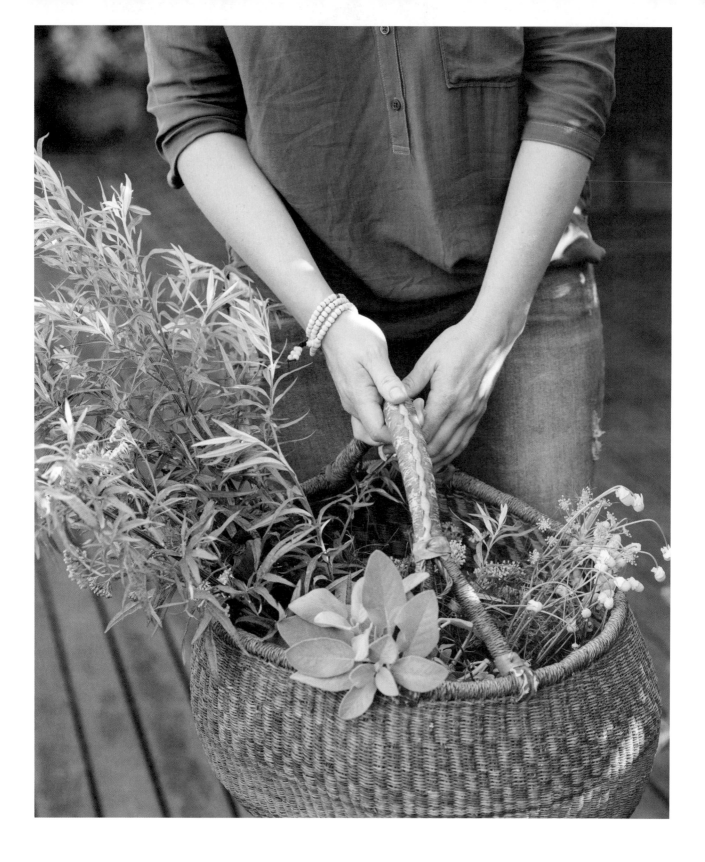

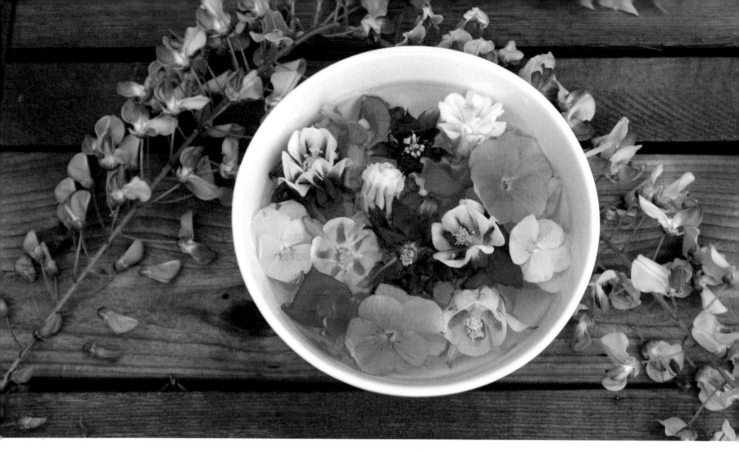

Flowers gathered in the spring and summer can be floated in a bowl of water where you will see them as you pass by.

OPPOSITE A roomy basket is nice to have for gathering garden goodies.

Day 3

GATHER GARDEN GOODIES

(ten minutes)

Grab a basket and shears and head out to the garden. No matter what time of year it is, try to find plants you can use indoors, whether in a bouquet, in a tea recipe, as a decoration, or on your altar. In the spring and summer, it may be flowers; in the summer and fall, vegetables and fruits; in the winter, twigs and leaves. You might consider focusing on plants that you want to learn more about and build your relationship with. As you gather the gifts of the garden, keep in mind the ethical harvesting guidelines mentioned earlier in the book: never take more than a third of the harvestable parts from a plant, ask for permission, and offer thanks to the plant. Indoors, arrange the gifts in a basket or bowl somewhere you will see them as you pass during the day.

Day 4

DESIGN A TEA OR MEDICINE JUST FOR YOU

(ten to thirty minutes)

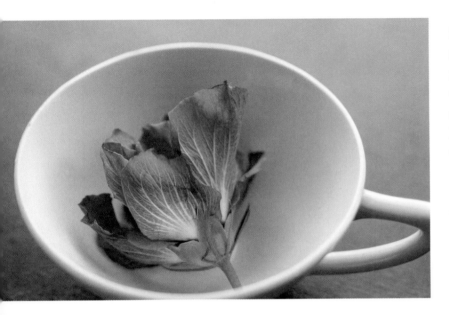

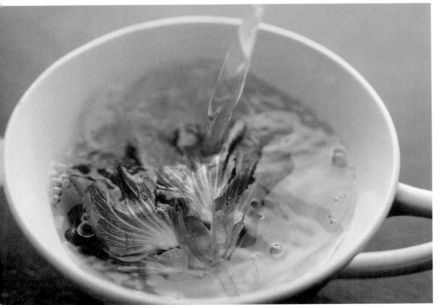

I love using fresh flowers like hibiscus to make tea. The flower quickly changes color as hot water is poured over it.

No matter what time of day it is, ask yourself: How do I feel? And how do I want to feel? It could be that you are stressed and want to relax, or you feel blue and need cheering up. There is a plant that can help you get there. Go to the last part of the "Plant Spirit Medicine" chapter and review the plant allies for specific needs. Choose one or two to make a tea with. If you don't have the plants on hand in your garden or pantry, now would be a good time to consider ordering plants for your garden or dried herbs for your apothecary. Once you've made your tea, drink and enjoy the benefits.

Alternatively or in addition, go back through the chapter "Fifty Sacred Plants for the Sanctuary Garden" and find one that you are growing. Spend some time studying it and finding recipes for the medicines it can make. These could be teas or tinctures or infused oils. Chances are you won't have to look far for the plant or the wisdom on how to use it. Just be sure to ask permission and thank the plant for its gifts when harvesting. For extra potency, make the medicine during the full moon.

Day 5

MAKE AN OFFERING TO A TREE THAT HAS SHARED ITS GIFTS

(ten minutes)

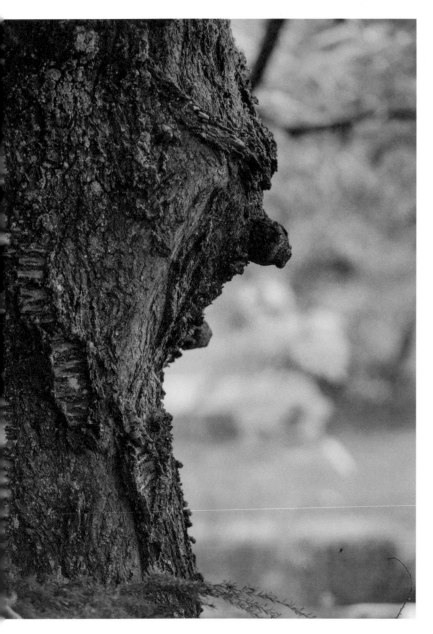

Making offerings is a way to acknowledge your gratitude for the abundant gifts of nature and to make wishes for peace in the world. You can adopt a practice of making offerings to trees that have given to you over the years, whether it be an ancient apple tree that has given fruit or a maple that had shared its shade and beauty. Find an old basket that you can leave out in the elements, or else create a little plate with a leaf or leaves placed on the ground or on an altar near the tree you want to honor. Place in it a few fresh flowers if available, a little rice, some incense, perhaps coins, some cornmeal, whatever you can think of that conveys gratitude. As you carefully arrange these offerings, breathe out the intention to create peace within yourself, in your neighborhood, and in your world. If you have more time, consider pruning or weeding around the tree to give it some extra love.

This elder cherry tree, named Wanda, has offered many gifts to her visitors, such as shade, beauty, memories, and habit.

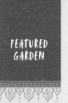

DAILY RITUAL *and* CEREMONY *in* BALI

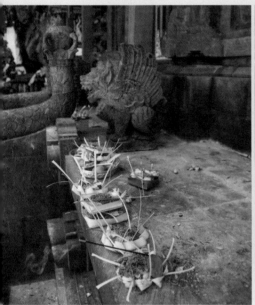 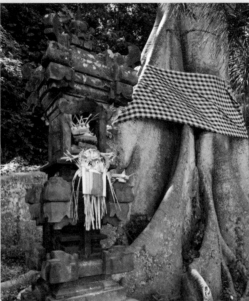 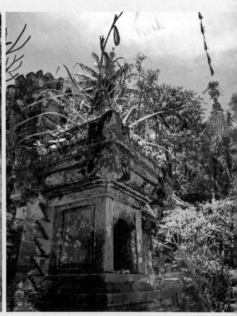

ABOVE, FROM LEFT TO RIGHT

Plants used in the daily offerings called *canang sari* have symbolic meanings and are grown in most home gardens.

Trees at temples wear black-and-white-checked cloths known as *saput poleng*, symbolizing dualities such as sorrow and joy.

Penjors line the streets during Galungan.

THE INDONESIAN ISLAND OF BALI, where the predominant religion is Hinduism, is populated by people who honor their interconnectedness with all of nature through ritual and ceremony. Plants are used for their symbolic and spiritual meanings in everything from simple offerings and blessings to elaborate festivals. Daily offerings called *canang sari*—small bowls woven from palm leaves and filled with plant parts—are placed outside of homes, in shrines, and at temples. Sacred spaces are everywhere and are highly respected by the culture, with specific etiquette to be followed. Trees are known to have spirits and, following

proper etiquette, are required to wear sarongs at temples, just like humans are.

During Galungan, an important Hindu holiday that occurs roughly every six months, the streets of Bali are lined by colorful penjors—tall bamboo poles decorated with coconut leaves and fruit, grains, flowers, and other plant parts, set up to the right of the entrance to each residence, along with a small bamboo altar bearing offerings. Galungan is a time to offer thanks to the creator of the universe, show devotion to the spirits of the ancestors, and celebrate the dominance of good over evil. Devotees pray and make offerings at the temples.

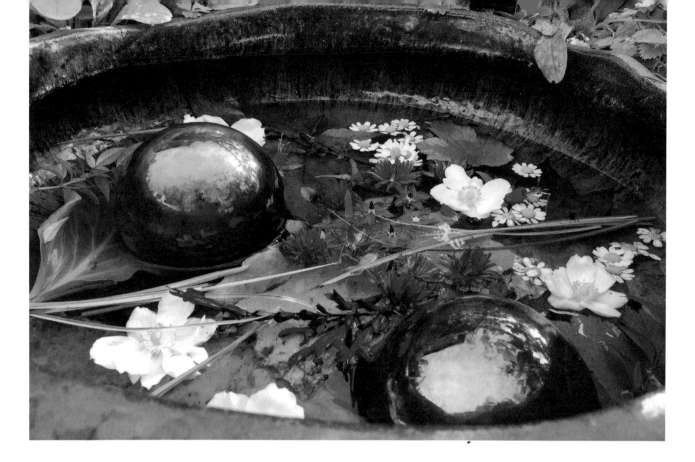

I use a simple water bowl at the entrance of my garden for botanical offerings every full and new moon, drawing on the plants in season at that time.

Day 6

JOURNAL ABOUT NATURE'S CYCLES

(ten minutes)

For five minutes, write down what you've noticed about the rhythms in nature and how they affect you. What is your favorite time of day? Do you enjoy watching the sun rise or set? Does the full moon give you powerful positive energy or does it cause you to drown in emotions? What is your favorite season? Your least favorite season?

Then take five minutes to add to your calendar some time slots to enjoy your favorite daily, monthly, and seasonal activities, especially at times you know you may need them the most. On the full moon, I take the entire day off and plan an energetic cleansing and ritual. Because I know I tend to get depressed in winter, I schedule time to be in the snow and at the spa.

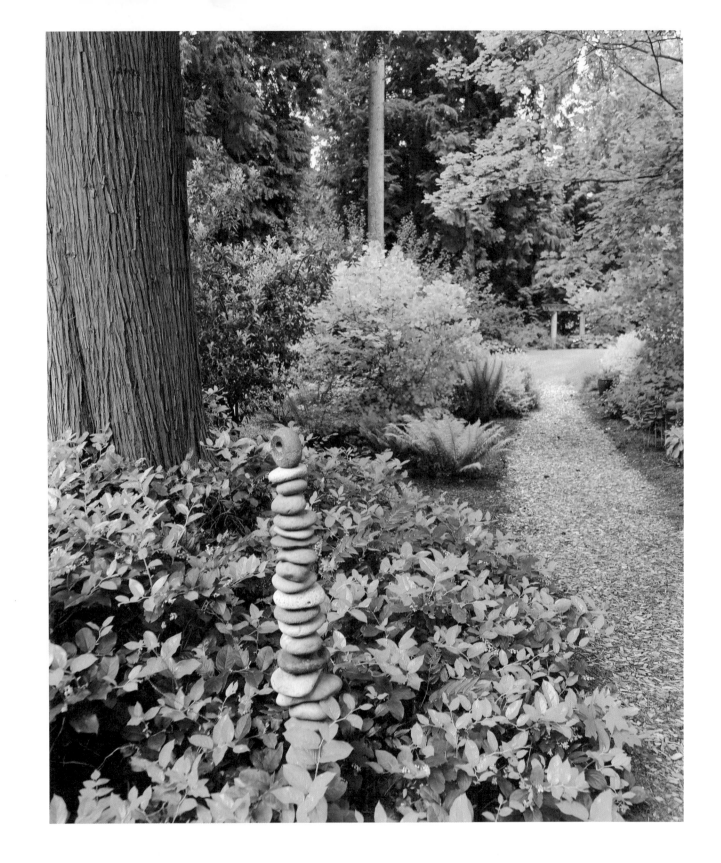

Day 7

PRACTICE A NEW PHYSICAL MOVEMENT

(ten to fifteen minutes)

Walking slowly with full attention is a way to bring yourself into your body and the present moment.

When we get stuck in our routines, it can often be hard to learn a new physical activity, but movement is so good for us! Choose a yoga pose, qigong movement, or stretches to do in the garden. You could even try something like hula hooping or using a kettlebell. Read an article or watch a video online first, and then if the weather is right practice it in the garden. You could also ask yourself what physical challenge most gets in the way of gardening for you. If it is a weak back, look at exercises that strengthen your core. If you have tight hips, find an exercise that stretches your hamstrings.

You can also try mindful walking, walking slowly with full attention as a way to bring yourself into your body and the present moment. You can do this even if it's raining or snowing out, as long as you dress appropriately. Choose a route to walk in your sanctuary. It doesn't need to be long; walking 10 feet and then turning around and walking back the same way, turning around and doing it again, is fine. Let your body take you for a walk at a pace of its choosing. Keep your eyes cast down to filter out visual input and place your attention in your legs and feet. Notice how the foot rolls from the heel to the ball of the foot to the toes; notice how walking is a process of losing balance and then finding it again. If you can walk barefoot on grass, notice the coolness and moisture under your feet. Breathe deeply and mindfully while you walk.

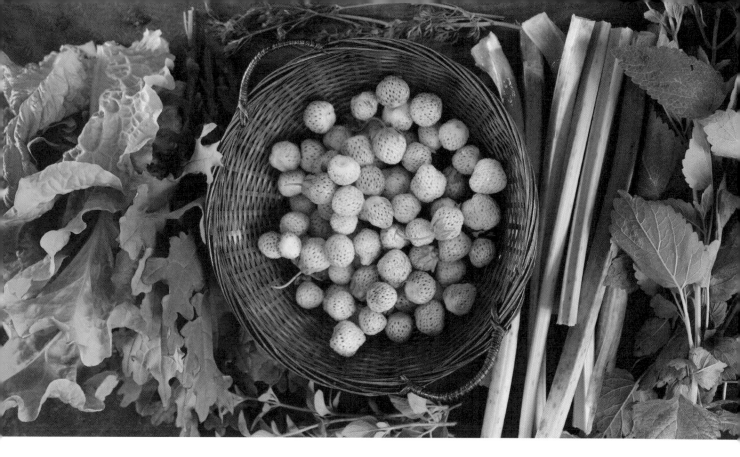

Day 8

CREATE A GRATITUDE RITUAL

(five minutes)

Science has shown that practicing gratitude is good for our health. On this day, spend five minutes feeling into what you are thankful for—even if the smallest things, such as "I'm thankful for this beautiful tree outside of my kitchen window" or "I'm grateful my son did his chores without being asked"—and creating a ritual to express the gratitude you feel. Taking this time could be as easy as doing a morning meditation in the shower, making a journal entry, or adding a symbolic item to an altar and saying a prayer. Sharing your gratitude with another is a way to amplify it, whether by writing a thank-you letter to someone who has impacted your life in a positive way or making a bouquet from the garden. Try to repeat this one as often as possible.

Day 9

EXCHANGE ENERGY WITH A TREE

(ten to thirty minutes)

Learning to feel the spirit of your plant allies and exchange energy with them is foundational to finding healing in your sacred space. This meditation will get you started.

1 Approach a tree you'd like to connect to. Imagine how the tree sees you. Imagine how it sees its environment and every other living being that comes to it—the birds, the insects, the roots of neighboring plants, people and other mammals. Ask permission of the tree to exchange energy with it.

2 Sit with your back against the trunk of the tree. Put both of your feet firmly and flat on the ground.

3 Take some focused deep breaths for thirty to sixty seconds. Inhale deeply, filling your chest and belly. Exhale out of your mouth. Continue breathing in this way.

4 With each breath, start to feel the pulse of the tree. Imagine the energy flowing from the tree's roots up through the trunk and into its canopy.

5 Focus your gaze on a leaf at the top of the canopy. Feel the sunlight

warming, radiating, and photosynthesizing in the tissues. Take that energy and move it downward into the rest of the tree and into your own body.

6 Breathe this energy in and out throughout your whole being, radiating, warming, and nourishing yourself. Do this for as long as you would like—and know that the tree is there to support you with this process. The tree is in no hurry and is always welcoming.

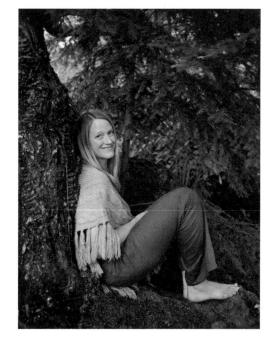

Exchanging energy with a tree can be instructive and soothing to the nervous system.

Day 10

CONDUCT A PERSONAL LETTING-GO CEREMONY

(fifteen to thirty minutes)

We all suffer loss in our lives, whether it is the loss of a loved one or relationship, or witnessing pain in the world around us. We tend to carry grief with us, and processing it can take time and space. A personal ceremony conducted in our sacred space can help us move through the stages of grief with more ease. Candles, incense, photos, letters, and other significant objects can be part of this ceremony. Here is a review of the steps:

1 Set your intentions.

2 Clean and clear the space.

3 Call in spiritual allies for support.

4 Do activities that move energy, such as burning slips of paper on which prayers have been written or using water to bless or release objects.

5 Wrap up with gratitude.

One of my favorite rituals to process grief is to say goodbye to the pain or person and list what I am grateful for and what I will miss. For example, my grandmother passed while I was writing this book, and in my personal ceremony I said, "Goodbye, Grandma. I will miss your laugh and sassiness, which was so fun to be around." You can do a ceremony several times at different stages of grief, and you might make a special tea or plant medicine to support you in this process.

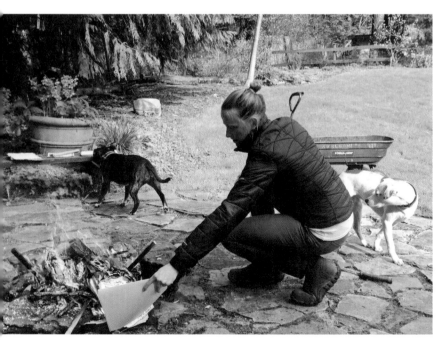

This letting-go ceremony involved burning documents.

Day 11

GET TO KNOW YOUR LEAST FAVORITE WEED

(ten minutes)

We all have a plant (or two or three) that makes gardening difficult. However, most "problem" plants have great potential, whether they are ecologically valuable, edible, medicinal, or hold a sacred power. Go into the garden and find your least favorite weed. Look at it through curiosity glasses: How can this plant benefit me instead of being a pain? Then read up about it.

You might also identify a small area to focus on and then spend ten minutes mindfully weeding that area, thanking each plant as you pull it up. With or without gloves, with or without a hand tool, grasp the plant at its base and loosen the soil around its roots if you can. Pull it out gently so as not to break off the roots, shake the soil off, and add it to your compost pile—or your green smoothie. Someone I know found purslane growing in her veggie beds, and when she learned about the nutrients it contains, she used it in her smoothie at lunch. I told her that before long she would be putting it in soups and salads, and on her face.

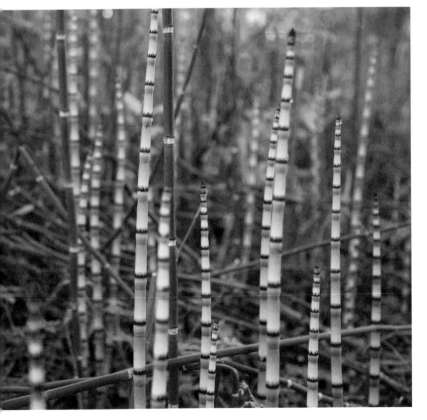

Though commonly known as a weed, horsetail has been used for medicinal purposes for centuries in many different cultures.

Day 12

BUILD OR ADD TO A CAIRN

(ten to fifteen minutes)

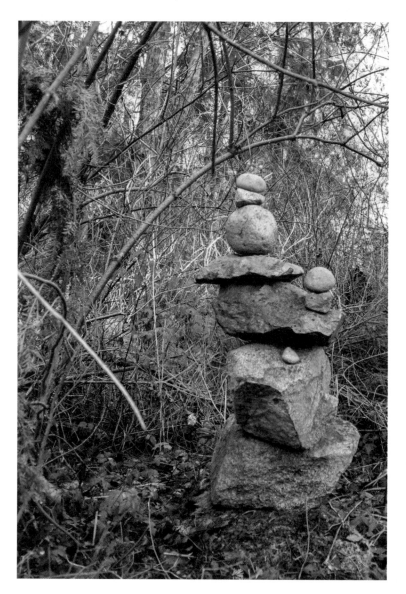

Building a cairn in your sacred space can be a meditative experience. First, find a flat and stable site to build on, such as a gravel bed, a stump, or a large stone. Collect a variety of sizes and types of stones from the site. I like to ask the stones, "Who wants to help with [state the intention]?" and see which stone or stones come to my attention. Then begin stacking stones so they are balanced on top of each other. Play with the stones. Turn them on their edges. Make sure they will not topple over if the wind blows or if a bird lands on them. This is a great activity for children who could use grounding or focus. My son says it is a good meditation for him.

After you have built a cairn, you can continue adding to it mindfully, one stone at a time. You might bring a stone back from somewhere you have traveled to or just from another corner of the garden. Hold an intention or say a prayer as you place it.

Building a cairn can be a meditation.

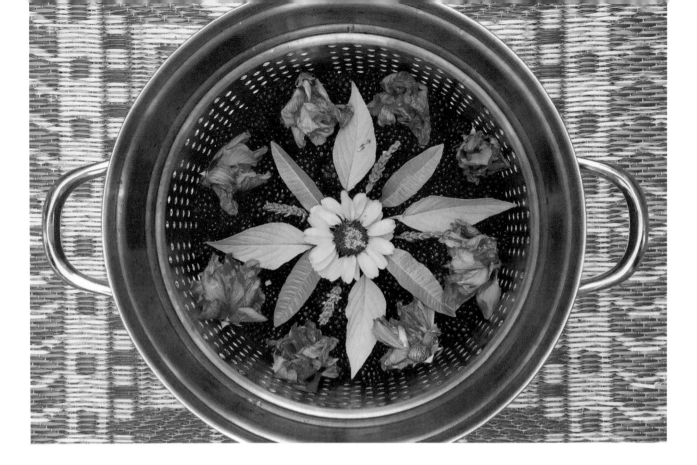

Create your mandala from materials such as blossoms and leaves.

Day 13

CREATE A MANDALA WITH PLANTS

(fifteen minutes)

First, find a space in your garden that feels right and is asking for a mandala to be built. This may be a small space you see regularly or one that is a little out of the way. Next, spend a few minutes gathering materials from the garden—leaves, twigs, seed heads, flowers, stones, and such. Then give yourself time to let the creative juices flow. Start in the center of the circle and build your design outward. It can be helpful to focus on one word—*abundance*, *joy*, *love*, or *peace*, for instance—as a prayer while you build.

Day 14

MEDITATE AND JOURNAL ON SUSTAINING SANCTUARY

(ten minutes)

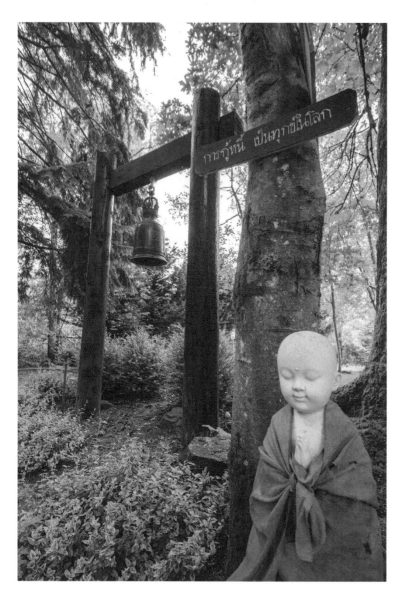

Get yourself grounded and seated for a quick meditation. For five minutes, focus on your sanctuary and what it will take to create what you want for yourself and maintain that. Are there things in your life that take up too much time and energy that you need to let go of and say goodbye to? Are there things you'd like to invite into your life? Then take five minutes to journal about your meditation, maybe drawing a picture or listing what you saw or felt.

Remembering to take the time to meditate on what we want in our lives is helpful in maintaining harmony and wellness.

We all need sanctuary—a place to get recharged, to get nourished, to feel whole and loved. Sanctuary can be found in the world around us, in our gardens, in our homes, in our workplace, and most important, within ourselves. It takes practice and it takes time to fully love ourselves and create environments that support us. This can often be difficult to do, especially if we have found ourselves in a life or a culture that doesn't acknowledge the need. I hope this book has gotten you started on the path to finding sanctuary and has encouraged you to realize you can get there moment by moment, anywhere you go.

After you have read this book, I suggest finding like-minded souls who you can do this work with. Ideally, you can encourage each other and hold space for each other in the process. Help each other garden, make tea, go to a yoga class together, make medicine together, and witness each other in a ceremony or with rituals. Read some books from the "Further Reading" list or perhaps take a class on something that was new and exciting in this book. The world is full of opportunities to make the most of your life. In creating your own sanctuary, always remember that you are both the author and the main character of your story. Blessings on your journey!

Ceremony and Ritual

Alexander, Jane. *The Smudging and Blessings Book: Inspirational Rituals to Cleanse and Heal.* New York: Sterling, 2009.

Farmer, Steven D. *Sacred Ceremony: How to Create Ceremonies for Healings, Transitions, and Celebrations.* Carlsbad, CA: Hay House, 2002.

Ingerman, Sandra. *Medicine for the Earth: How to Transform Personal and Environmental Toxins.* New York: Three Rivers Press, 2000.

Herbs and Herbalism

Breedlove, Greta. *The Herbal Home Spa: Naturally Refreshing Wraps, Rubs, Lotions, Masks, Oils, and Scrubs.* North Adams, MA: Storey, 1998.

Cech, Richo. *Making Plant Medicine*, 4th edition. Williams, OR: Herbal Reads, 2016.

de la Forêt, Rosalee. *Alchemy of Herbs: Transform Everyday Ingredients into Foods and Remedies That Heal.* Carlsbad, CA: Hay House, 2017.

Edwards, Victoria H. *The Aromatherapy Companion.* North Adams, MA: Storey, 1999.

Foster, Steven, and Rebecca Johnson. *Desk Reference to Nature's Medicine.* Washington, DC: National Geographic Society, 2006.

Gladstar, Rosemary. *Rosemary Gladstar's Medicinal Herbs.* North Adams, MA: Storey, 2012.

Grieve, Margaret. *A Modern Herbal*, two volumes, revised edition. New York: Dover Publications, 1971.

Groves, Maria Noel. *Body into Balance: An Herbal Guide to Holistic Self-Care.* North Adams, MA: Storey, 2016.

Hartung, Tammi. *Cattail Moonshine and Milkweed Medicine.* North Adams, MA: Storey, 2016.

Hobbs, Christopher, and Leslie Gardner. *Grow It, Heal It: Natural and Effective Herbal Remedies from Your Garden or Windowsill.* New York: Rodale, 2013.

Keville, Kathi. *The Aromatherapy Garden: Growing Fragrant Plants for Happiness and Well-Being.* Portland, OR: Timber Press, 2016.

Kloos, Scott. *Pacific Northwest Medicinal Plants.* Portland, OR: Timber Press, 2017.

Pursell, J. J. *The Herbal Apothecary.* Portland, OR: Timber Press, 2015.

Sonoma Press. *Do-It-Yourself Herbal Medicine: Home-Crafted Remedies for Health and Beauty.* Berkeley, CA: Sonoma Press, 2015.

Sonoma Press, *Essential Oils and Aromatherapy: An Introductory Guide.* Berkeley, CA: Sonoma Press, 2014.

Wood, Matthew. *The Earthwise Herbal Repertory: The Definitive Practitioner's Guide.* Berkeley, CA: North Atlantic Books, 2016.

Massage

Finando, Donna, and Steven Finando. *Trigger Point Therapy for Myofascial Pain: The Practice of Informed Touch.* Rochester, VT: Healing Arts Press, 2005.

Lidell, Lucinda. *The Book of Massage: The Complete Step-by-Step Guide to Eastern and Western Techniques.* New York: Simon and Schuster, 2001.

Movement

Pearlman, Barbara. *Gardener's Fitness: Weeding Out the Aches and Pains.* Lanham, MD: Taylor Trade Publishing, 1999.

Mushrooms

Arora, David. *Mushrooms Demystified,* 2nd edition. Berkeley, CA: Ten Speed Press, 1986.

Cotter, Trad. *Organic Mushroom Farming and Mycoremediation: Simple to Advanced and Experimental Techniques for Indoor and Outdoor Cultivation.* White River Junction, VT: Chelsea Green, 2014.

Fischer, David W., and Alan E. Bessette. *Edible Wild Mushrooms of North America: A Field-to-Kitchen Guide*. Austin, TX: University of Texas Press, 1992.

Stamets, Paul. *Growing Gourmet and Medicinal Mushrooms*, 3rd edition. Berkeley, CA: Ten Speed Press, 2000.

———. *Mycelium Running: How Mushrooms Can Help Save the World*. Berkeley, CA: Ten Speed Press, 2005.

Nature Therapy

Jayne, Tabitha. *The Nature Process: Discover the Power and Potential of Your Natural Self and Improve Your Well-Being*, 2nd edition. TNP Press, 2017.

Louv, Richard. *The Nature Principle: Human Restoration and the End of Nature-Deficit Disorder*. Chapel Hill, NC: Algonquin Books of Chapel Hill, 2011.

Nutrition

Nickerson, Brittany Wood. *Recipes from the Herbalist's Kitchen*. North Adams, MA: Storey, 2016.

Plant Spirit

Amaringo, Pablo. *Ayahuasca Visions*. http://protocole-oracle.com/DIVERS/Ayahuasca_Visions_Pablo_Amaringo.pdf

Blair, Katrina. *The Wild Wisdom of Weeds*. Mad River Junction, VT: Chelsea Green, 2016.

Buhner, Stephen Harrod. *The Secret Teachings of Plants: The Intelligence of the Heart in the Direct Perception of Nature*. Rochester, VT: Bear & Company, 2004.

———. *Sacred Plant Medicine: The Wisdom in Native American Herbalism*. Rochester, VT: Bear & Company, 2006.

Chase, Pamela Louise, and Jonathan Pawlik. *Trees for Healing: Harmonizing with Nature for Personal Growth and Planetary Balance*. North Hollywood, CA: Newcastle, 1991.

Graves, Julia. *The Language of Plants*. Great Barrington, MA: Lindisfarne Books, 2012.

Mann, A. T. *The Sacred Language of Trees*. New York: Sterling Ethos, 2012.

Wohlleben, Peter. *The Hidden Life of Trees*. Vancouver, Canada: Greystone Books, 2016.

Planting in Layers

Bloom, Jessi, and Dave Boehnlein. *Practical Permaculture for Home Landscapes, Your Community, and the Whole Earth*. Portland, OR: Timber Press, 2015.

Falk, Ben. *The Resilient Farm and Homestead: An Innovative Permaculture and Whole Systems Design Approach*. Mad River Junction, VT: Chelsea Green, 2013.

Reynolds, Mary. *The Garden Awakening: Designs to Nurture Our Land and Ourselves*. Cambridge, England: Green Books, 2016.

Weaner, Larry, and Thomas Christopher. *Garden Revolution: How Our Landscapes Can Be a Source of Environmental Change*. Portland, OR: Timber Press, 2016.

Rain Gardens

Woelfle-Erskine, Cleo, and Apryl Uncapher. *Creating Rain Gardens: Capturing the Rain for Your Own Water-Efficient Garden*. Portland, OR: Timber Press, 2012.

Sacred Space

Kavasch, E. Barrie. *The Medicine Wheel Garden*. New York: Bantam Books, 2002.

McDowell, Christopher Forrest, and Tricia Clark-McDowell. *The Sanctuary Garden: Creating a Place of Refuge in Your Yard or Garden*. New York: Simon and Schuster, 1998.

Minter, Sue. *The Healing Garden: A Natural Haven for Emotional and Physical Well-Being*. London: Headline Book Publishing PLC, 1993.

Murray, Elizabeth. *Cultivating Sacred Space: Gardening for the Soul*. Rohnert Park, CA: Pomegranate, 1997.

Pettis, Chuck. *Secrets of Sacred Space*. St. Paul, MN: Llewellyn Publications, 1999.

Silf, Margaret. *Sacred Spaces: Stations on a Celtic Way*. Orleans, MA: Paraclete Press, 2001.

Woods, Pamela. *Gardens for the Soul*. London: Conran Octopus Ltd., 2002.

Wildlife Habitat

Xerces Society. *Gardening for Butterflies*. Portland, OR: Timber Press, 2016.

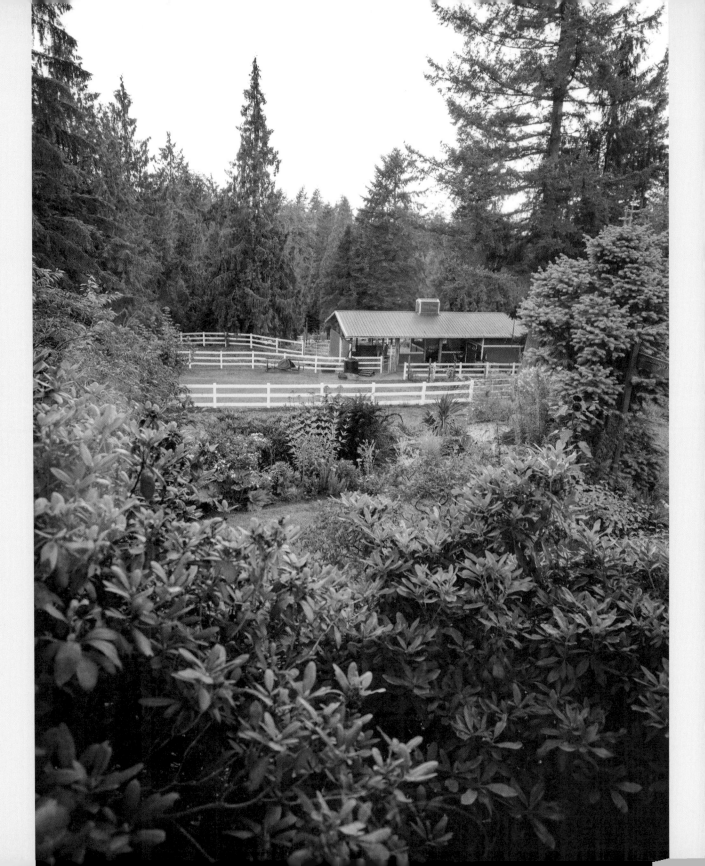

ACKNOWLEDGMENTS

Writing this book was not a solo journey—it has involved many individuals as well as sacred spaces. I couldn't have written this book without the support of my sons, Micah and Noah, who tagged along on road trips and photo shoots, becoming curious historians and talented photographers in their own right.

To all of my teachers, mentors, and friends over the years, especially while this book was being conceived and birthed—sincere gratitude for the support and lessons I have received through a difficult period in my life. My mom, Susan McKinley; father, David Bloom; plus friends, guides, and teachers: Tenney Kerr, Thalia Ryer, Jason Foster, Jesse Goldmark, Mark Edwards, Lacia Lynn Bailey, Nunutsi Otterson, Jack Beeching, Erin Verginia, Caleb Mardini, Zac Kopra, Angie and Doug Van Pelt, Amber Comes, Andrew Millison, Patricia Foreman, Peter Nguyen, Katie Vincent, Erin Merrihew, Sandra Ingerman, and Casey Stewart.

To my incredible editors, the shapers of this book, much love—to Juree Sondker, who championed the idea, bringing it to life, and to Lorraine Anderson, whose tremendous help and kindness in keeping me on track made this book possible. To Shawn Linehan and Patrick Barber, thank you for the creative lens and the beauty you brought to the book. Thanks to all of the folks at Timber Press for trusting me with an idea and for bringing this book into the world.

To all of the lovely folks with land they have stewarded that was photographed for this book—thank you for opening up your sacred spaces to help inspire others to develop their own vision and dream of their own sacred spaces.

And to the plants, animals, and stones, all of the givers—thank you for always being safe for me to learn from. I look forward to a lifetime of continual love and connection with all of you.

INDEX